# Small Animal Pain Management

# Small Animal Pain Management

Gwendolyn L. Carroll, MS, DVM, DACVA

Department of Small Animal Medicine and Surgery

College of Veterinary Medicine

Texas A&M University

Many thanks to the AAHA Press Editorial Advisory Board:
Dr. Laurel Collins, ABVP
Dr. Richard Goebel
Dr. Charles Hickey
Dr. Clayton McKinnon
Dr. Richard Nelson, ABVP
Dr. Hal Taylor

AAHA Press
12575 W. Bayaud Avenue
Lakewood, Colorado 80228



ISBN 0-941451-69-0

# Contents

# Preface

*Small Animal Pain Management* was written with the busy practitioner in mind. Although veterinarians can manage a patient with pain in many different ways, the intent of this text is to provide veterinarians with options so that no patient need go untreated. For practitioners who currently use limited analgesics and analgesic techniques in their practices, I have provided basic information that I hope will be easy to follow, useful, and reliable. The information provided can be used the first day the book is consulted. For practitioners who currently rely heavily on analgesics and analgesic techniques in their practices, I have provided information on new analgesics and analgesic techniques that may complement the drugs and techniques already employed. The text necessarily reflects my bias. The dosages I have provided without reference are those that I use daily. As in any case management, clinical judgment must be used to individualize treatment for any given patient.

I have limited the references that I have cited to those that are particularly helpful, those that provide specific drug dosages or techniques that I do not normally employ, and those that provide recent new evidence of the efficacy of analgesics or analgesic techniques. The interested reader should consult these references. This text is intended to be a quick reference and is not intended to replace chapters and journal articles or more complete previously published texts such as: Short, C.E., and van Poznak, A. (eds.), *Animal Pain* (Publisher: Churchill Livingstone).

# Acknowledgments

I would like to acknowledge the contribution that my patients have made to my understanding of their treatment needs. I am indebted to Drs. Bernie Hansen and Lizette Hardie for sharing with me their insight regarding pain management when I was learning how to be an empathetic caregiver. I would also like to thank Drs. Pete Hellyer and Sandee Hartsfield for their continued support of my professional development.

Ms. Jan Worley receives my appreciation for the line drawings, Mr. Steve Walenta for many of the photographs (Figures 2-1 A, 3-4 A-D, 3-5, 6-2, A-1 A, A-1 D, A-1 G-J), and Mr. Peter Erling for his technical assistance with the manuscript. I also appreciate the thoughtful review of my manuscript by the peer reviewers, and editorial staff, particularly Ms. Mary Kay Kozyra, at AAHA.

Lastly, a special thanks to my family, Ms. Frances Currie, and Mr. Tim Carroll for their patience in this and all endeavors.

# Chapter 1 Identifying the Patient with Pain

One of the greatest impediments to effectively treating patients with pain is recognizing the pain. It is important to identify patients with pain. Once the veterinarian has determined the degree of pain being expressed by the patient, he or she can select the appropriate treatment and monitor the treatment's success.

## Definition of Terms

Terms such as stress, distress, and pain are often used interchangeably in veterinary medicine. Stress occurs when external or internal factors change an animal's equilibrium.[1] Distress, which results from an inability to respond to stress, reflects a mental or physical state caused by fear, anxiety, or pain.[2] Acutely, distress is decreased by tranquilization, but chronically, a change in the environment or behavior is required.[2] Tranquilization is a state in which the patient is relaxed and indifferent to its surroundings and to minor pain[2] (e.g., IV catheterization). Anxiety is an uneasiness or apprehension of impending danger, and may be accompanied by restlessness. The term "suffering" is generally avoided; suffering has emotional connotations (perhaps implying victimization), which are generally not helpful in addressing patients with pain.

There are several definitions for *pain* in human literature. The International Association for the Study of Pain proposed the most common definition for acute pain: "Pain is an unpleasant sensory and emotional experience associated with actual or potential tissue damage or described in terms of such damage."[3] Pain involves an injury and awareness of the injury, and results in behavioral or biological change. One can characterize pain as superficial (skin, subcutaneous tissue), deep (muscle, bones, joints, and attachments), visceral, or psychogenic.[2] Based on onset and duration, pain can be classified as acute or chronic. Perioperative pain is generally acute, even if imposed on a chronically painful animal. Recognizing and treating acute vs. chronic pain are different issues, require different assessments, and will be discussed separately.

In nonverbal patients, it is difficult to distinguish between the behavioral and physiologic responses caused by stress and those caused by pain. Although the responses may be similar, the treatments are different. It is equally important to control both distress and pain, since they impact directly on each other (i.e., pain and anxiety are linearly related). For example, in humans, a preoperative interview with an anesthesiologist that alleviates apprehension decreases the amount of postoperative analgesic required by 50%.[4] Anecdotally, in veterinary anesthesia, patients seem to recover in the same way that they were induced (e.g., a rough induction is usually followed by a rough recovery). A "stress-free" induction and a quiet, calm recovery are desirable. The role of tranquilizers will be discussed in chapter 3.

## Pain Pathways

Without doubt, individuals respond variably to pain. In people, differences in psychological factors, levels of endogenous opioids, and receptor responses probably contribute to individual variability.[4] In order to understand pain responses and therapeutic alternatives, it is important to have a basic understanding of pain physiology. In 1965, Melzack and Wall proposed that pain could be modulated in the spinal cord and brain to impact pain perception (gate theory).[4] Descending modulation explained psychological influences and centrally acting analgesics. Initial modulation occurs in the spinal cord's dorsal horn, which contains several laminae where nociceptive input is processed.[5] Spinal modulation at the level of the substantia gelatinosa is believed to involve two populations of opioid receptors, a noradrenergic system, a serotonergic system, possibly a GABA-ergic system (GABA is γ-aminobuteric acid), and substance P.[4] Relay cells in lamina I–V synapse with ascending nociceptive fibers.[5] Ascending afferents are believed to produce physical aspects of pain via the thalamus to the cerebral cortex with ascending afferents to the limbic system, producing the emotional aspects of pain.[4]

Peripheral nociceptors are afferents that, after stimulation, transmit nervous impulses to the CNS.[6] Nociceptive afferents may be small myelinated Aδ neurons, large myelinated Aβ fibers, or unmyelinated C fibers.[5] Some mechanisms may increase or decrease the sensitivity of peripheral nociceptors. Tissue damage stimulates the inflammatory cascade, resulting in the conversion of arachadonic acid into metabolites that cause hyperalgesia. Physical stimulation (pressure, heat, or chemicals), circulatory and pH changes, norepinephrine release (efferent activity), prostaglandin synthetase (cyclooxygenase), serotonin, substance P, and bradykinin may change receptor activity.[4]

Development of peripheral pain may be interrupted by blocking the sympathetic nerves (e.g., local anesthetics);[4] by inhibiting phospholipase, which is the catalyst for conversion of phospholipids to arachadonic acid (e.g., steroids); by inhibiting lipoxygenase, which uses arachadonic acid to produce the leukotrine inflammatory mediators; or by inhibiting cyclooxygenase, which converts arachadonic acid to endoperoxide (e.g., nonsteroidal anti-inflammatory drugs [NSAIDs]).[5] NSAIDs also function in other ways: Aspirin inhibits the release of bradykinin from damaged tissue[5] and carprofen's mode of action is believed to be other than cyclooxygenase or 12-lipoxygenase inhibition.[7] There is evidence of peripheral opioid receptors, and researchers are examining the use of opioids in peripheral tissues.

Because afferent fibers ascend or descend at least three segments before synapsing in the substantia gelatinosa,[4] reflex activity may be able to modulate pain. Nociceptive impulses from the viscera and body surfaces converge on the same neurons in the substantia gelatinosa, which may lead to viscero-somatic, viscero-sympathetic, viscero-visceral, and somatic-visceral reflexes.[4]

To summarize current analgesic therapies, opioids inhibit afferent nociceptive impulses at the brain and spinal cord, local anesthetics directly interrupt neural-impulse conduction, and NSAIDs prevent the nociceptor sensitization that accompanies inflammation.[8] Therapy is discussed in more detail in chapter 4.

## Techniques for Identifying Patients with Pain

Most veterinarians determine the presence of pain by looking at a combination of factors: their expectations regarding a given surgery, a patient's physiological response, and a patient's behavioral response. Even if veterinarians do not consciously examine patients for pain, assessing each patient's comfort is an inherent component of their evaluation. Veterinarians examine patients to determine if their disease is improving (e.g., better use of a limb after orthopedic surgery) or deteriorating (e.g., worsening signs of pancreatitis). Part of the assessment involves evaluating the patient's comfort level; usually, an increase in comfort is associated with an improvement of the disease process. In this chapter, the focus will be on the criteria that veterinarians use to make such assessments.

Veterinarians bring some bias to their evaluation of pain in animals. It is important that as caregivers, veterinarians recognize this bias. Some veterinarians say that they did not appreciate how painful surgical intervention could be until they had surgery themselves. Veterinarians expect some surgical procedures to cause their patients minimal discomfort. Many veterinarians have observed, for example, that an ovariohysterectomy causes only a slight disruption of normal activity, based on how well patients appear to tolerate the procedure. However, an objective evaluation of ovariohysterectomies in dogs indicates that it is a noxious and fatiguing experience.[9]

Why have veterinarians perceived ovariohysterectomies to be benign? One reason relates to how dogs behave when they interact with people: Dogs are very social and generally have a heightened awareness during hospitalization. Their increased alertness and activity may obscure their demonstration of pain behaviors when they interact with clinic staff. Dogs that are videotaped after an ovariohysterectomy appear to engage in more normal activity when they interact with clinic staff and in more pain behaviors when they are left alone (unpublished observation). The veterinarian may not appreciate discomfort in a client's animal unless he or she is familiar with its normal behavior. When a veterinarian's own pet undergoes the same procedure, the veterinarian is better able to appreciate subtle behavioral differences postoperatively. Pet owners, therefore, are in a good position to determine if their pet is painful. This has been demonstrated in client-owned cats undergoing onychectomies (unpublished observations). The owners' reports of their cats' lameness accurately reflected which cats were receiving an analgesic and which were receiving a placebo (unpublished observations). It is important for practitioners to actively solicit owners' opinions about their pets' postoperative behavior when they are monitoring analgesic therapy.

## Expectations Regarding the Degree of Pain from Different Surgical Procedures

Having acknowledged that veterinarians have some bias, what surgeries are expected to be painful? Recently, more people agree that if a surgery is painful in humans it is likely to be painful in dogs and cats (with any exceptions resulting from the fact that dogs and cats are quadrupeds and humans are bipeds). People are recognizing that procedures such as ovariohysterectomies are painful in animals. Veterinarians are also able to draw on their experience of how patients have tolerated various procedures. For example, practitioners originally grouped ear surgeries with procedures that might cause pain but that were not intensely painful, based on early pain literature suggesting that ear surgeries were not very painful. After they observed how several dogs recovered from ablations of the ear canal, however, it became apparent that such patients are painful and are difficult patients to manage postoperatively. These patients also seem to require more inhalant anesthetic (higher vaporizer settings) during surgery and more intraoperative opioids than most surgical patients (e.g., most fracture repairs and exploratory laparotomies). Such findings are consistent with those found with severe pain-inducing procedures. It is possible that ear ablations are particularly painful because the tissue is chronically inflamed. But the difference in how patients tolerate aural-hematoma repair and how poorly they tolerate ear ablations indicates that one cannot necessarily lump procedures together based on anatomic location.

Examples of surgeries that veterinarians expect to be extremely painful are full limb amputations and thoracotomies (particularly median sternotomies). Other surgeries that are expected to be painful are those associated with extensive tissue trauma (e.g., a fractured femur). Cranial abdominal procedures are moderately painful. Other procedures, such as surgery for distichiasis, are probably only mildly painful, but may be irritating or annoying to the patient. For a more complete list of procedures and medical conditions and the anticipated level of pain, refer to Table 1-1.

Patients that undergo elective procedures and exploratory laparotomies invariably experience more pain postoperatively than preoperatively. However, a patient's comfort may be improved after undergoing procedures that stabilize or correct a preexisting abnormality (e.g., a closed reduction of a metacarpus). It is also reasonable to expect that the amount of surgical time and trauma may impact how much pain the procedure causes the patient. For a particular surgical procedure, an inexperienced surgeon may induce a different amount of tissue trauma from that produced by a surgeon experienced in gentle tissue handling. Similarly, if an extensive amount of muscle or soft tissue is traumatized during tissue handling, one can expect that the patient will experience more discomfort than occurs with minimal trauma to muscle and soft tissue.

The inherent danger in using only expectations to determine which patients will be painful is that veterinarians may misinterpret a pet's response to a painful stimulus. Veterinarians should make allowances for individual differences in pain perception. If veterinarians expect a procedure to be relatively minor and a patient behaves otherwise, the inclination is to think that the pet is anxious or disconcerted for reasons other than pain. It is important to remember that

***Table 1-1.*** *Categories of surgical procedures and medical conditions by anticipated level of pain. These classifications are not meant to be used to deny any patient analgesic therapy. The level of pain is only an approximation; some animals may be more painful than anticipated.*

| Irritating (annoying) and/or mildly painful | Mildly painful to moderately painful | Moderately to severely painful | Severely painful |
|---|---|---|---|
| Dried blood | Endoscopy with biopsy | Localized burns or ulcerations | Extensive burns or ulcerations |
| Urine scald | Dental cleaning/ extraction | Corneal ulcerations | Bile peritonitis |
| Clipper burns | Tracheotomy | Enucleation | Pancreatitis |
| Intravenous catheterization | Arterial catheterization | Mandibulectomy | Total hip replacement |
| Distended bladder | Muscle biopsies | Thoracic or lumbar disc surgery | Cervical disc surgery |
| Repaired aural hematoma | Aural hematoma | Onychectomy | Rhinotomy |
| Superficial lacerations | Stabilized fractured radius/ulna or tibia/ fibula | Stabilized fractured femur or humerus, or pelvis | Forelimb or hindlimb amputation |
| Some perirectal procedures | Castration | Mastectomy | Ear ablation |
| Eyelid procedures (entropion, distichiasis) | Caudal abdominal procedures (cystotomy, ovariohysterectomy) | Cranial abdominal procedures (diaphragmatic hernia, GDV) | Thoracotomy (especially sternal splits) |

background or environment, purpose, age, training, breed, and sex may influence how an animal responds to pain. Some animals may tolerate procedures better than others. If an animal is injured during competition, the injury may go unnoticed as both hunting trials and sled dog competitions have demonstrated. The animals are working, and may not recognize their injury until after the competition. For a simpler example, consider the three-legged lame dog that becomes sound when pursuing a squirrel. With respect to age, puppies respond to vaccination procedures differently than adult dogs. Puppies may become alarmed at their first injection, yelping and squirming; adult dogs are generally more tolerant, often not flinching or vocalizing when the veterinarian injects them. Additionally, dogs respond to vaccinations differently based on their breed and the relationship they have to their owners. Whether the dog lives inside or outside, whether it is a companion or a working dog, and whether it has been socialized all contribute to how painful—or even how threatening—a vaccination will be. Another example is the small dog that requires a toenail clipping. If the dog has been hurt in the past during a nail clipping, it may vigorously resist this relatively benign procedure. The dog may not even allow a veterinarian to examine its feet.

Increasing amounts of evidence suggest that males and females perceive and respond to pain and analgesics differently. Dog trainers report that males and females take correction as well as tolerate discomfort differently. Certainly in studies of human pain, researchers are realizing how the sexes differ in their reaction to pain. In an investigation of young men and women undergoing extraction of wisdom teeth, women were far more responsive to kappa agonists administered for pain than were men, even when the women had significantly more pain preoperatively.[10] Different responses to analgesics by males and females have bearing on the use of analgesics, since past studies on analgesia may not have represented the sexes equally.

## The Physiologic Responses of Patients Experiencing Pain

Pain is a stressor, and many of the responses to pain or to stress will be the same. How patients respond to pain is discussed in this section (see Table 1-2); the physiologic responses to stress are covered in chapter 2. Physiologic changes in response to chronic pain may be subtle and may reflect a decreased well-being. In chronic pain, the pituitary-adrenal axis is hyperactive. The physiologic changes that patients with acute pain experience are similar to those that occur in response to catecholamines. The responses include tachycardia, hypertension, arrhythmias, peripheral vasoconstriction, increased respiratory rate, and changes in body temperature. The physiologic response to other stressors may mimic those in response to pain. For example, tachycardia is compatible with pain and fear. Additionally, there are similar physiologic responses to metabolic conditions other than pain; anemic animals or hyperthermic animals may be tachycardic. Blood loss may produce a tachycardia mediated through hypovolemia. Physiologic responses to drugs may also mimic

*Table 1-2. Physiological manifestations of acute pain.*

| System | Manifestation |
|---|---|
| Cardiovascular | Increased blood pressure and heart rate; vasoconstriction |
| Pulmonary | Increased respiratory rate; splinting |
| Nervous | Dilated pupils |
| Digestive | Loss of appetite; possibly vomiting, diarrhea; evacuation of anal glands; salivation; constipation |
| Musculoskeletal | Tense muscles, abnormal posture, muscle tremors |
| Immune | Decreased resistance; stress leukogram; possible increase in metastasis |
| Neuroendocrine | Increased catabolism; decreased anabolism |

pain responses. Administering perioperative drugs such as acepromazine may precipitate hypotension and a reflex tachycardia (hypotension is generally not a problem in healthy patients that are receiving low preanesthetic doses). Similarly, administering anticholinergic or inotropic drugs may produce tachycardia. The veterinarian should examine the differentials for the tachycardia and institute treatment (e.g., if hypotension is suspected, the administration of intravenous fluids may lower the patient's heart rate); initiating analgesic therapy is not warranted based on a single physiologic change.

When a veterinarian is evaluating physiologic responses, a difficult clinical situation occurs when a patient is actually "shocky" as a result of pain. The heart rate is elevated, the mucous membranes are pale, the respiratory rate is rapid, and the respiratory pattern is shallow. The patient's mental status may be obtunded. Resolving the situation requires very careful evaluation of the patient's physiologic status. In addition to administering fluids and stabilizing the affected body systems, veterinarians should include analgesics as part of the treatment plan if the etiology is pain. Similarly, critically ill patients with serious medical or surgical abnormalities may experience a significant degree of pain concurrently. Caregivers worry about doing harm by administering analgesics. However, the added stress of pain may cause these patients to decompensate. Many reliable analgesics are available for veterinarians to use safely in patients they are monitoring. Monitoring the painful patient is discussed in chapter 5.

Clinically, it is probably not realistic to use endocrine changes to evaluate patients for pain. Historically, neurally derived factors (e.g., epinephrine, norepinephrine, vasopressin, substance P, and calcitonin-gene-related peptides) that respond quickly to a stressor, and endocrine-derived factors (e.g., adrenocorticotropic hormone, β-lipoprotein, β-endorphin, cortisol, prolactin, growth hormone, glucagon, insulin, renin-angiotensin, aldosterone, pituitary thyroid axis, and pituitary gonadal axis hormones) that respond more slowly and last longer have been used to evaluate acute stressors.[11] Veterinarians have used cortisol,[12–18] glucose,[18] and catecholamines[19–21] to evaluate stressors and analgesic therapy in dogs and cats.

Patients that experience chronic stressors often demonstrate hyperactivity of the pituitary-adrenal axis; the dexamethasone-suppression test and the corticotropin releasing factor test may be useful in identifying long-term efficacy of therapeutic intervention in patients with chronic pain.[11] In such patients, there is also evidence that serotonin is presynaptically depleted (increased turnover).[22]

There is a large amount of individual variation in these stress-related hormones and metabolites, and it may be difficult to distinguish the responses from surgery, drugs, and pain. It is important to remember that there is no set neuroendocrine response to stress. The central nervous system activates various neuroendocrine responses to stress; the conditions under which individuals respond are dynamic and can be modified by intrinsic and extrinsic factors.[11] Although individuals respond differently to stress, there is a real metabolic cost to unrelieved pain. The increased levels of catabolic hormones and decreased levels of anabolic hormones that occur in patients that are painful[23] are discussed in chapter 2.

## Behavioral Signs in Painful Patients

Behavioral signs alone may not identify painful patients. Obtunded patients may be unable to demonstrate behavioral signs. Similarly, patients that are

*Table 1-3. Behavioral responses to pain and outwardly recognizable physical characteristics consistent with pain.*

| Behavioral response | Dogs | Cats |
|---|---|---|
| Vocalization | Groan, whine, whimper, growl | Groan, growl, purr |
| Facial expression | Fixed stare, glazed appearance | Furrowed brow, squinted eyes |
| Body posture | Hunched; prayer position; laterally recumbent | Generally sternal |
| Self-awareness (guarding and self-mutilation) | Protects wound or limb, limps, or fails to bear weight; licks and chews wounds and surgical sites; rubs area | Protects wound or limb, limps, or fails to bear weight; licks and chews wounds and surgical sites |
| Activity | Restless or restricted movement; trembling (shivering) | Restricted movement; may see stereotypies (i.e., repeated meaningless movements such as circling) |
| Attitude: socialization and comfort seeking | Increased aggression or timidity (fearfulness) | Comfort seeking or hiding; may see aggressiveness |
| Appetite | Decreased | Decreased |
| Urinary and bowel habits | Increased urination; failure in house training; urinary retention | Failure to use litter box |
| Grooming | Loss of sheen in hair coat, particularly in chronically painful dogs | Failure to groom, particularly in chronically painful cats |
| Response to palpation | Protecting, biting, vocalizing, withdrawing, orienting | Protecting, biting, scratching, vocalizing, withdrawing, orienting; escape |

exhausted or heavily sedated may be unable to demonstrate behavioral signs. By the time the veterinarian has recognized the behavioral signs of pain, the patient has exhausted many of its coping mechanisms. The reason for this is that there is little evolutionary advantage to demonstrating pain behaviors. An animal that draws attention to itself when ill or injured may become prey or at least be challenged in social-group ranking. Additionally, some physical attributes may be outward signs of pain (e.g., a poor hair coat) and are easy to recognize. These physical attributes are not necessarily specific for pain; for example, a poor hair coat may reflect inadequate nutrition, a failure to groom, or increased metabolic stress. Recognizable physical attributes of pain and stress are discussed later in this chapter.

Behavioral signs are somewhat species specific; for example, primates have more control over their facial muscles and thus have more expressive faces. People have long believed that cats are more stoic than dogs,[24] and that they respond to pain differently than do dogs.[24,25] Detecting chronic pain in cats is perhaps more challenging than identifying it in dogs, but acute pain is generally readily recognizable (e.g., a kitten's failure to bear weight after an onychectomy). Without doubt, cats are treated for pain less frequently than are dogs. In a recent survey[25] to identify analgesia use, only 1 of 15 cats received analgesics postoperatively, but failure to recognize pain was not the reason. It may be that cats suffer silently. Common behavioral signs in painful patients are discussed in the following paragraphs (see Table 1-3).

**Vocalization**

Vocalization is probably the easiest sign of pain and distress to recognize—it is the one characteristic that invariably guarantees patients receive treatment in my hospital's intensive care unit and intermediate care ward. The patients may have different surgical procedures, medical conditions, surgeons, primary clinicians, technicians, and anesthesiologists, but all patients that vocalize are examined and with few exceptions are treated with analgesics, sedatives, and/or tranquilizers. Conversely, patients that suffer quietly may be denied treatment. As stated earlier, there is no evolutionary advantage for animals to vocalize when they are painful, so a patient must have exhausted its coping mechanisms if it resorts to vocalization.

There are several different types of vocalization. Painful dogs may groan, whimper, whine, or growl; barking is uncommon in the painful animal, but may occur when the animal is distressed or anxious. Painful cats (although they are less likely than dogs to vocalize) may growl, purr, groan, or (uncommonly) meow. It is unfortunate for cats that purring is usually associated with comfort since it may be misinterpreted in the painful animal. There are certainly occasions in which dogs and cats vocalize when they are not painful. For example, animals may vocalize because they are dysphoric during recovery from anesthesia; confined animals in strange surroundings may vocalize due to

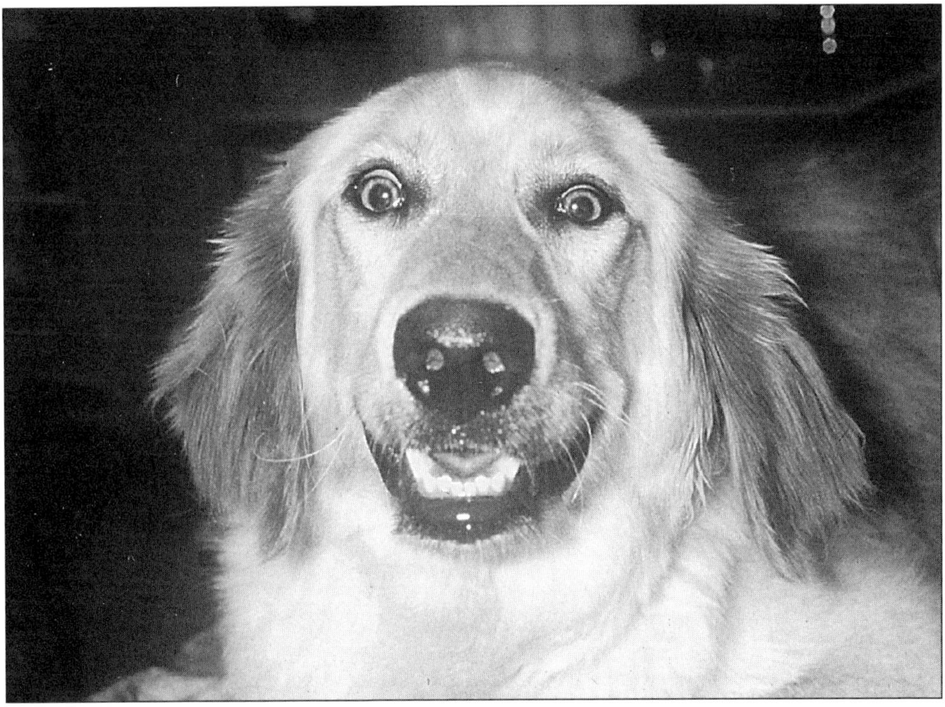

*Figure 1-1. The wide-eyed facial expression of this Golden Retriever indicates that it is excited; additionally, the dog is salivating.*

distress. The practitioner should evaluate and treat all of these conditions appropriately.

**Facial Expression**

Facial expression may be very enlightening when evaluating a patient. Although dogs and cats are limited in what their facial muscles will allow them to do, veterinarians assess both the physical and mental status of dogs and cats every day by looking at their faces. With practice, veterinarians are generally able to distinguish a dog that is anxious from a dog that is painful. The Golden Retriever in Figure 1-1 has a wide-eyed expression and is salivating. This particular dog will benefit from tranquilization. Painful dogs often have a fixed stare with dilated pupils and their eyes appear glazed. It is unlikely that the facial expression of the cat in Figure 1-2 would be misinterpreted. The cat will benefit from tranquilization. Painful cats also have expressive faces; they furrow their brows and squint, as illustrated in Figure 1-3.

**Postural Changes**

Postural changes often occur when an animal experiences uncontrolled pain. For example, it is easy to

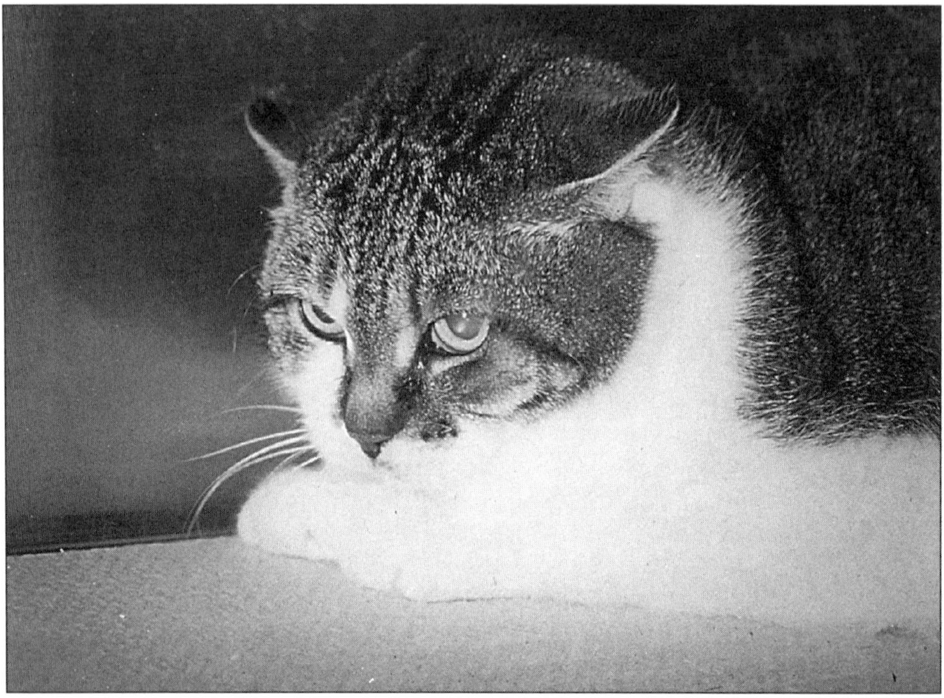

***Figure 1-2***. *Most veterinarians recognize that the intent of this cat is to aggressively avoid interacting with a caregiver. Notice the flattened ears. (Photograph courtesy of Dr. Sandee Hartsfield.)*

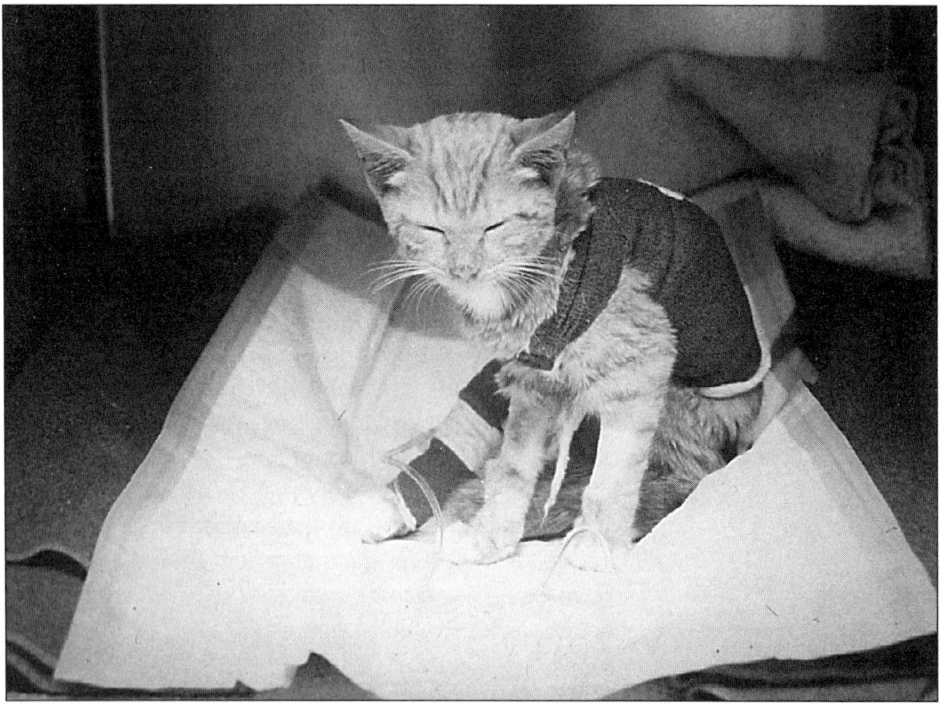

***Figure 1-3***. *The furrowed brow, squinting eyes, and flattened ears of this cat are easily recognizable as painful signs in this post-thoracotomy cat.*

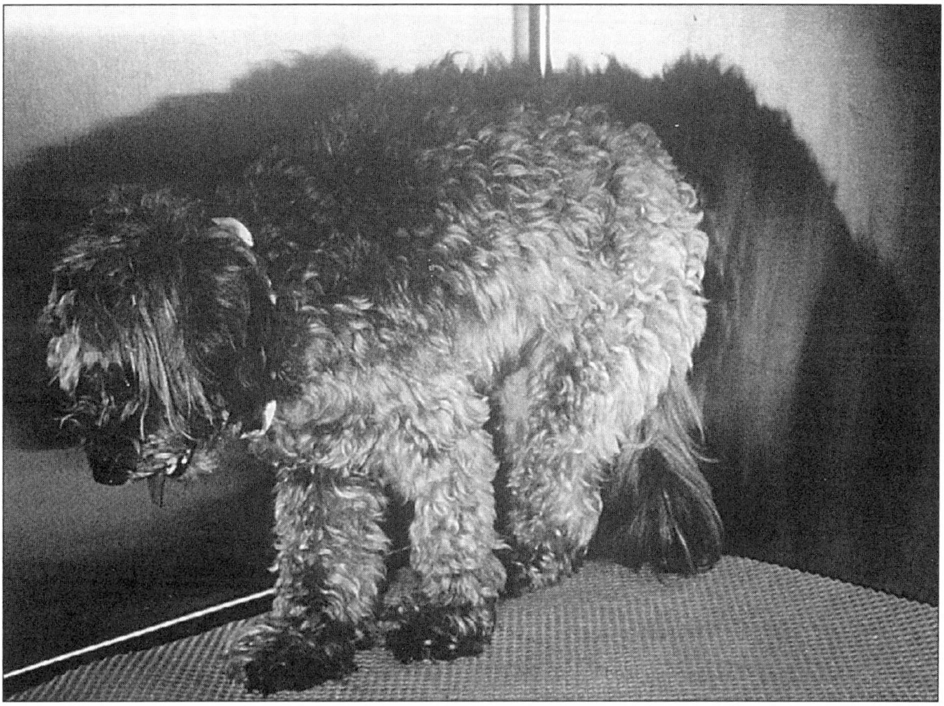

*Figure 1-4*. *This dog has cervical disc disease. Notice the arched back and lowered head. The dog's eyes follow movement, but he does not turn his head.*

recognize the posture of a dog with cervical disc disease. The dog's back is arched and the head is lowered (see Figure 1-4). Generally, the dog will follow you with its eyes, but will not move its head. These dogs may salivate more than normal. The dog in Figure 1-5 has a presumed infection of a lumbar disc ($L_4$). The dog presented with a history of weight loss and a poor hair coat, and snapped when it was petted along the back. While the veterinarian was discussing the dog's case with the owner, the dog assumed the prayer position (see Figure 1-5) several times. The owner reported that the dog commonly assumed this position. The classic prayer position should not be confused with the "play bow" that dogs demonstrate. The prayer position is generally assumed when the animal has cranial abdominal pain. In the case of the dog in Figure 1-5, the position seemed to alleviate his discomfort, perhaps by decreasing pressure on the spine.

The cat in Figure 1-3 was recovering from a thoracotomy and maintained this position for several hours. It appeared that the cat was trying to sleep. Every time

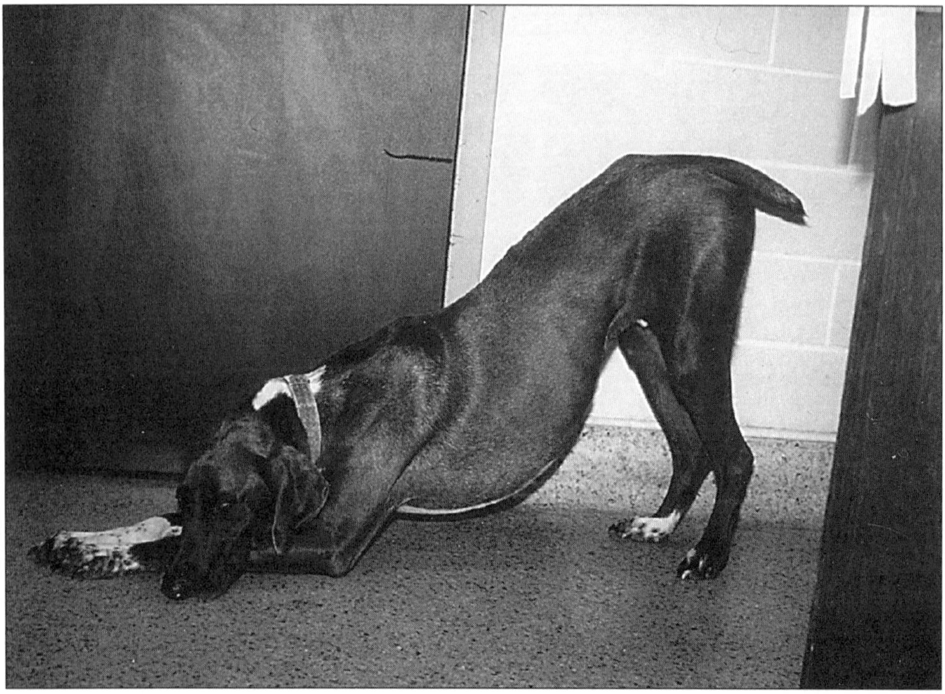

***Figure 1-5**. This dog had a presumed infection of $L_4$ and assumed the "prayer position" regularly.*

the cat's head fell, it startled and sat up. Dogs and cats may spend extended amounts of time in positions that are protective, even at the expense of sleep.

**Self-Awareness (Guarding and Self-Mutilation)**

Just as posture may be protective after thoracic or abdominal surgery, patients may isolate and protect wounds on limbs. Patients will limp or refuse to use a limb that is painful; patients will withdraw an affected limb from palpation. Surgical and traumatic wounds may also precipitate self-mutilation. Patients may lick, chew, or bite at wounds. After surgery, dogs spend more time licking.[26] Self-mutilation may also occur with nerve injury.

**Personality and Activity**

Changes in personality may be associated with pain or stress. After surgery, dogs will greet their caregivers less frequently.[26] A friendly animal may become aggressive. Similarly, a timid and fearful animal may seek comfort; although this is less likely, it does occur, particularly in cats. The animal's activity level may change; a painful animal may become restless, seemingly unable to get comfortable. Likewise, a normally active animal may resist attempts to remove it from its cage, or it may refuse to move at all. Painful or stressed dogs often tremble. Cats frequently hide, distancing themselves from their human and feline companions.

**Appetite**

Changes in appetite are fairly reliable indicators of discomfort. In a study of onychectomized cats, appetite was a good indicator of which animals received an analgesic and which received a placebo (unpublished observations). A painful animal may refuse to eat entirely, may eat less than normal, may be enticed to eat only with special foods, or may have to be hand fed. To objectively determine the appetite of a chronically hospitalized animal, it may be helpful to examine how much weight the patient has lost.

**Urinary and Bowel Habits**

Changes in an animal's toilet habits may also indicate pain. Dogs may urinate more frequently; previously housebroken dogs may urinate and defecate in inappropriate places; constipation may occur. If painful, cats may fail to use their litter boxes, often urinating in their beds.

**Grooming**

In painful animals that are marginally coping, behavioral signs may be subtle. Although not specific for pain, one of the most reliable signs in chronically painful cats is an unkempt appearance; cats stop grooming (see Figure 1-6). In dogs, the hair coat may lose its sheen. Although not a behavioral indicator of pain, it is an outwardly recognizable sign.

The absence of behavioral signs does not mean that a patient is pain free. To determine the best treatment for a patient, veterinarians should look not only at how much pain they anticipate a surgical or medical condition will cause, but also at the patient's physiologic and behavioral responses. To assist veterinarians when they are evaluating painful dogs and cats, some institutions provide a "Pain Score Evaluation Form" that assigns scores to behaviors and physiologic variables.[27] In the beginning of one's career, it is easy to spend a great deal of time in front of cages watching animals and doing physical examinations to determine if a patient is painful. As a veterinarian gains more experience, though, he or she will need to spend less time assessing patients. If a practitioner is not sure

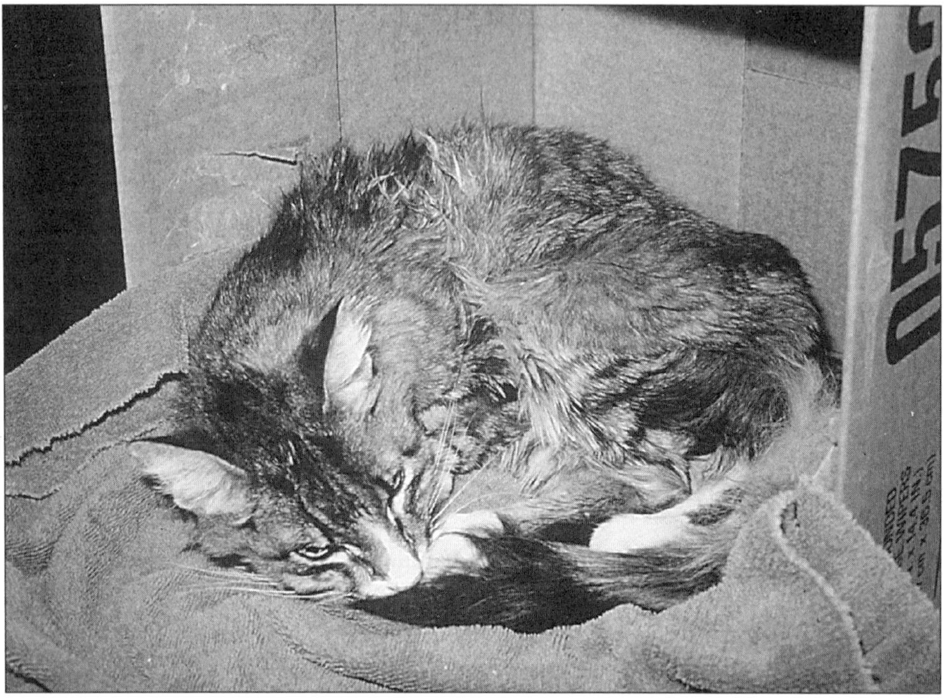

***Figure 1-6***. *Notice the unkempt appearance of this cat.*

whether or not the patient is painful, it is advisable to proceed with treatment. After treatment, the patient's response should be reevaluated. It is not necessary to treat the patient again if it does not show improvement after receiving the appropriate therapy.

## References


1. Committee on Pain and Distress in Laboratory Animals, Institute of Laboratory Animal Resources, Commission on Life Sciences, National Research Council. Recognition and alleviation of pain and distress in laboratory animals. Washington: National Academy Press, 1992:1–9.
2. Wright EM, Marcella KL, Woodson JF. Animal pain: evaluation and control. Lab Animal 1985; 14:20–35.
3. International Association for the Study of Pain. Report of the International Association for the Study of Pain Subcommittee on Taxonomy. Pain 1979; 6:249–52.
4. Cousins MJ. Management of postoperative pain. In: Proceedings of the International Anesthesia Research Society, 60th Congress. Las Vegas: International Anesthesia Research Society, 1986: 32–39.
5. Potthoff A, Carithers RW. Pain and analgesia in dogs and cats. Compendium Continuing Educ Practicing 1989; 11:887–97.
6. Sackman JE. Pain: Its perception and alleviation in dogs and cats. Part 1. The physiology of pain. Compendium Continuing Educ Practicing 1991; 13:71–79.

7. Mathews KA. Nonsteroidal antiinflammatory analgesics to manage acute pain in dogs and cats. Compendium Continuing Educ Practicing 1996; 18:1117–23.

8. Lee VC, Rowlingson JC. Pre-emptive analgesia: update on nonsteroidal anti-inflammatory drugs in anesthesia. In: Advances in anesthesia, vol. 12, St. Louis: Mosby, 1995:69–110.

9. Fox SM, Mellor DJ, Lawoko CRO, Hodge H, Firth EC. Effects of different combinations of halothane, butorphanol, and ovariohysterectomy on behavior in the dog. Proceedings of the twenty-second annual meeting of the American College of Veterinary Anesthesiologists. San Diego: American College of Veterinary Anesthesiologists, 1997:36.

10. Gear RW, Miaskowski C, Gordon NC, Paul SM, Heller PH, Levine JD. Kappa-opioids produce significantly greater analgesia in women than in men. Nature Medicine 1996; 2:1248–50.

11. Hargreaves KM. Neuroendocrine markers of stress. Anesth Prog 1990; 37:99–105.

12. Popilskis S, Kohn DF, Laurent L, Danilo P. Efficacy of epidural versus intravenous morphine for post-thoracotomy pain in dogs. J Vet Anaesth 1993; 20:21–25.

13. Day TK, Pepper WT, Tobias TA, Flynn MF, Clarke KM. Comparison of intra-articular and epidural morphine for analgesia following stifle arthrotomy in dogs. Vet Surg 1995; 24:522–30.

14. Fox S. Changes in plasma cortisol concentrations before, during and after analgesia, anaesthesia and anaesthesia plus ovariohysterectomy in bitches. In: Animal pain and its control, Proceedings 226 in conjunction with the Chapter of Anaesthetics & Intensive Care of the Australian College of Veterinary Scientists. Sydney: Post Graduate Committee in Veterinary Science University of Sydney, 1994:87–99.

15. Hansen BD, Hardie EM, Carroll GS. Physiological measurements after ovariohysterectomy in dogs: what's normal. Appl Anim Behav Sci 1997; 51:101–9.

16. Stobie D, Caywood DD, Rozanski EA, et al. Evaluation of pulmonary function and analgesia in dogs after intercostal thoracotomy and use of morphine administered intramuscularly or intrapleurally and bupivacaine administered intrapleurally. Am J Vet Res 1995; 56:1098–1109.

17. Hendrix PK, Raffe MR, Robinson EP, Felice LJ, Randall DA. Epidural administration of bupivacaine, morphine, or their combination for postoperative analgesia in dogs. J Vet Med Assoc 1996; 209:598–607.

18. Buback JL, Boothe HW, Carroll GL, Green RW. Comparison of three methods for relief of pain after ear canal ablation in dogs. Vet Surg 1996; 25:380–85.

19. Lin HC, Benson GJ, Thurmon JC, Tranquilli WJ, Olson WA, Bevill RF. Influence of anesthetic regimens on the perioperative catecholamine response associated with onychectomy in cats. Am J Vet Res 1993; 54:1721–24.

20. Benson GJ, Wheaton LG, Thurmon JC, Tranquilli WJ, Olson WA, Davis WA. Postoperative catecholamine response to onychectomy in isoflurane-anesthetized cats: effect of analgesics. Vet Surg 1991; 20:222–25.

21. Rawlings CA, Tackett RL, Bjorling DE, Arnold TH Jr. Cardiovascular function and serum catecholamine concentrations after anesthesia and surgery in the dog. Vet Surg 1989; 18:255–60.

22. Fishbain DA, Cutler R, Rosomoff HL, Rosomoff RS. Chronic pain-associated depression: antecedent or consequence of chronic pain? A review. Clin J Pain 1997; 13:116–37.

23. Benedetti C, Bonica JJ, Bellucci G. Pathophysiology and therapy of postoperative pain: a review. In: Benedetti C, Chapman CR, Moricca G, eds. Advances in pain research and therapy (vol 7). Raven Press, New York, 1984:373–407.

24. Crane SW. Perioperative analgesia: a surgeon's perspective. J Am Vet Med Assoc 1987; 191:1254–57.

25. Hansen B, Hardie E. Prescription use of analgesics in dogs and cats in a veterinary teaching hospital: 258 cases (1983–1989). J Am Vet Med Assoc 1993; 202:1485–94.

26. Hardie EM, Hansen BD, Carroll GS. Behavior after ovariohysterectomy in the dog: what's normal? Appl Anim Behav 1997; 51:111–28.

27. Hellyer PW, Gaynor JS. Acute postsurgical pain in dogs and cats. Compendium Continuing Educ Practicing Vet 1998; 20:140–53.

patients undergoing major surgery of the extremities also appears to be related to inadequate analgesia.[4]

Surgical and medical care of veterinary patients has improved greatly in the last several years. Veterinarians are currently able to perform complicated surgery and provide advanced medical care, which prolong life in patients that previously would have died or been euthanized. Caregivers should improve such patients' quality of life as well as extend their lives.

Clinically, it appears that sick patients that are kept comfortable and are minimally stressed recover sooner than patients that are allowed to experience unmitigated painful procedures and diseases. Although there are few such studies in dogs and cats, in an investigation of women undergoing laparoscopic tubal ligation, the best predictor of return to normal activity was the amount of pain the women experienced during the immediate postoperative 7-day period.[6] In veterinary patients treated for pain, there are limited objective measurements of improvement that might substantiate the reports of improved outcome in pain-free people. Currently, few well-controlled investigations of outcome evaluate hospital stay, morbidity, owner satisfaction, and recovery in animals with and without analgesic therapy. One such study, which examined behavior after an ovariohysterectomy, indicated a more rapid return to normal behavior in oxymorphone-treated dogs.[7] A study in rats[8] indicated that administering buprenorphine, an opioid analgesic, could reduce the detrimental effects of abdominal surgery on food and water consumption. In an investigation that examined the outcome in cats following onychectomy, about 28% more of the cats receiving postoperative butorphanol ate during hospitalization, compared to the cats receiving a placebo; 22% more of the cats receiving butorphanol ate during the first day at home, compared to cats receiving a placebo (unpublished observations).

Even without much published information regarding improved outcome, the attitude in veterinary teaching hospitals surrounding the use of analgesics has gradually changed. Clinicians of many disciplines often request analgesic therapy or consultations regarding

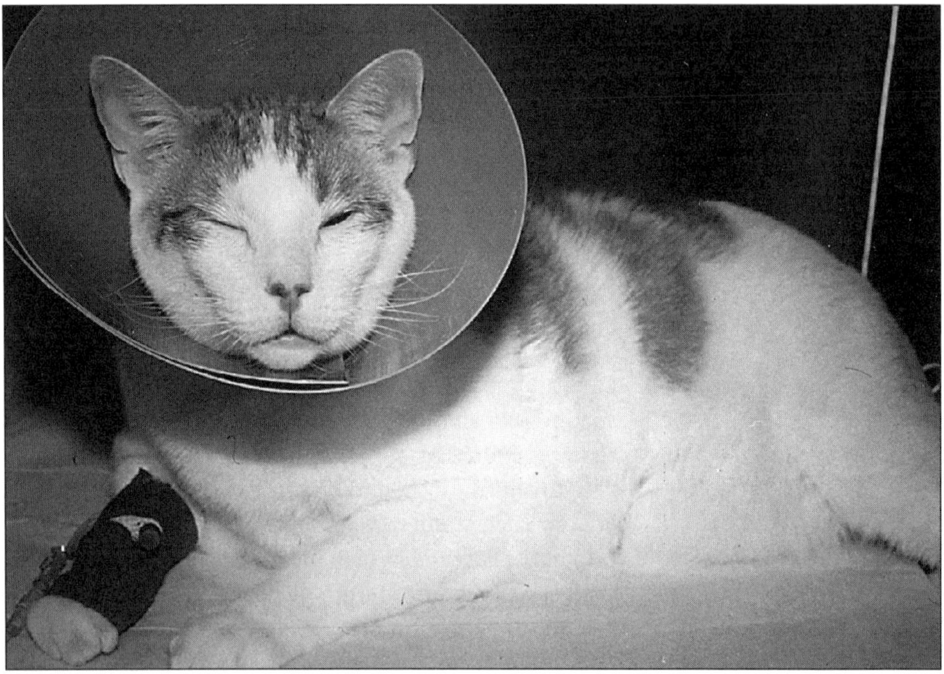

***Figure 2-1***. *An adult male castrated cat was operated on to correct subcutaneous urine spillage from a previous perineal urethrostomy. The cat received analgesia by a morphine epidural that the veterinarian administered after induction and prior to surgery to repair the surgical site. His appetite and attitude improved postoperatively.*
***Figure 2-1 A***. *Preoperatively, the cat shows no interest in his surroundings. Notice his facial expression.*

the use of analgesics in their patients. In addition to having gained a heightened awareness of the physiologic cost of unrelieved pain, clinicians recognize that patients do in fact regain normal functions (e.g., eating, drinking, grooming) sooner if pain is controlled during the perioperative period (see Figures 2-1 A to 2-1 C) or during the acute phase of a painful medical disease.

Another reason that analgesics are underprescribed is that veterinarians are often unable to accurately identify painful patients. Several scoring systems have been developed[9–11] and guidelines have been published[12–15] for recognizing pain. Systems have been based on physiologic and hormonal responses,[16–18] metabolites,[19] behavior,[9,14] and combinations of physiologic responses and behaviors.[11,20] Behavioral scoring systems (e.g., the visual analog scale, numerical rating scale, simple descriptive scale) have been recently

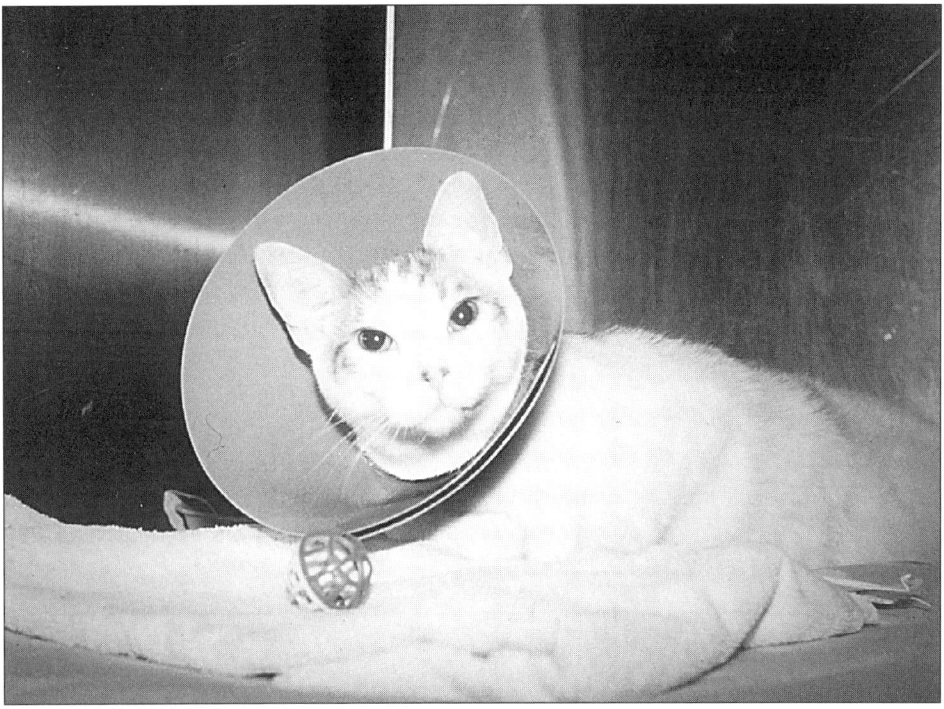

***Figure 2-1 B.*** *Approximately 16 hours after surgery, the cat was still comfortable, and appeared alert and interested in his surroundings.*

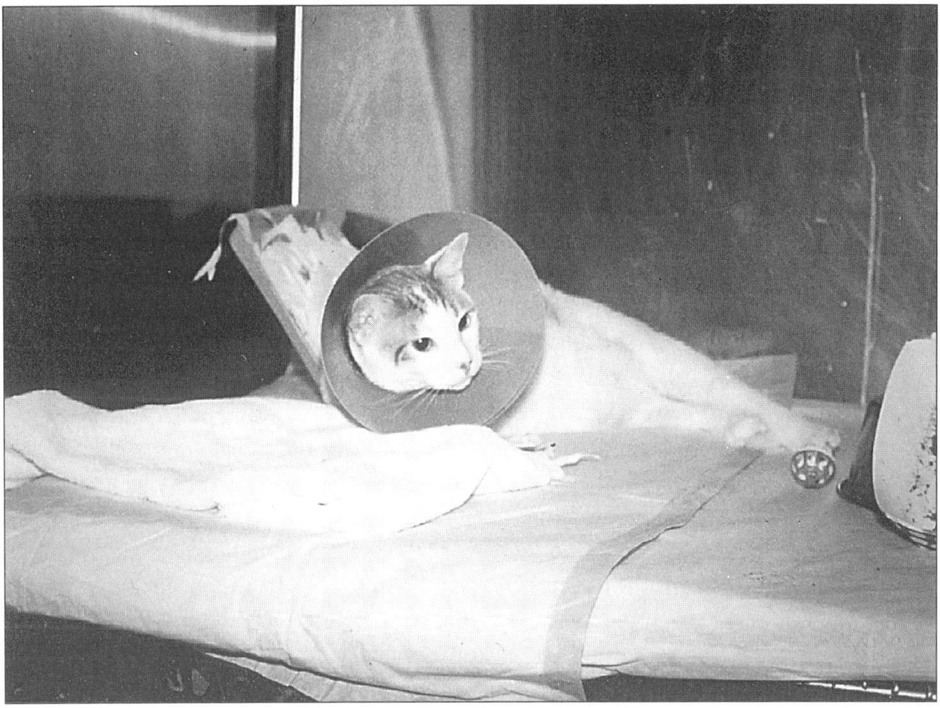

***Figure 2-1 C.*** *Additionally, he had a good appetite (notice the empty food bowl).*

compared.[21] Researchers have also examined in dogs the agreement between objective and subjective measures of postoperative pain and have found only a weak association.[22] Similarly, in cats, researchers found very little agreement when comparing postoperative hormonal and physiologic (excepting cortisol and indirect systolic blood pressure measurement) indicators of pain.[16] A practical solution that allows veterinarians to identify painful patients (discussed in chapter 1) is use of a combination of behavioral responses, physiologic responses, expectations regarding the amount of pain to be experienced from a surgery or medical condition, and the response to therapy. In the absence of clear evidence that small animal patients are not painful, it is unreasonable for veterinarians to withhold treatment for medical and surgical conditions that are painful in people.

## Importance of Pain Management

Several real physiologic costs are associated with unrelieved pain. Pain and fear can activate the stress response.[23] During the first 48 hours of a stress response, changes in cardiac output, increases in oxygen consumption, vasoconstriction, hypothermia, decreased urine output, changes in insulin concentration, and immunologic impairment may occur; between 2 and 5 days, patients may become hypermetabolic, developing a negative nitrogen balance.[23] During this period, cardiac output, oxygen consumption, and regional blood flow all increase. Additionally, hyperthermia, proteolysis, gluconeogenesis, ureagenesis, and glucose intolerance may develop.[23] The endocrine response to trauma or surgery is an increase in catabolically active hormones (catecholamines, cortisol, adrenocorticotropic hormone [ACTH], antidiuretic hormone [ADH], glucagon, and aldosterone) and a decrease in anabolically active hormones (insulin, testosterone).[4] The endocrine response results in increases in blood glucose, plasma cyclic AMP, free fatty acids, ketone bodies, and blood lactate; additionally, metabolism and other activators of the stress response such as oxygen consumption increase.[4] Veterinarians aggressively treat dehydration, hypovolemia, infection, hypoxemia, and temperature changes (other activators of the stress response), but do not treat fear or pain. Recovering from an acute injury has been compared to running a marathon every day. The physiologic demands are great, but if the patient is provided with analgesia and a stress-free environment, the patient's physiologic responses can be improved. Indeed, in people, a stress-free perioperative period is known to be beneficial.[24]

## Complications of Untreated Pain

Postoperative complications that result from pain-induced pulmonary dysfunction have already been addressed. Pain-induced complications are also associated with major-joint surgery (e.g., hip, knee). Persistent postoperative pain and limitation of movement impair normal muscle metabolism, causing muscle atrophy and delaying a return to normal function.[4] Pain-induced anxiety causes cortically mediated increases in blood viscosity and promotes clotting, fibrinolysis, and platelet aggregation, possibly potentiating thromboembolic disease.[4]

Pain alters the immune system and may be immunosuppressive.[25] Intriguing recent evidence indicates that pre- and postoperative morphine analgesia attenuates a surgically induced increase in metastasis in rats.[25] Providing adequate analgesia should be a minimum standard because immunosuppression resulting from pain promotes pathology that the immune system would usually resist.[25]

## The Caregiver's Responsibility

Clients expect that their pets will receive optimal care in a veterinary facility. It is common for clients to inquire about which analgesics will be provided. Veterinarians are sworn to decrease pain and suffering (Veterinarian's Oath). Veterinarians have historically withheld analgesics because they perceived that it was in the patient's best interest. However, excellent and safe analgesics are available today, and sufficient evidence documents that analgesics are advantageous. Additionally, it is now clear that patients do not benefit from experiencing pain. As veterinarians have access to excellent methods for monitoring the physiologic responses of their patients receiving analgesics, there is little reason to withhold therapy.

How long should the practitioner provide analgesia? After an onychectomy, cats receiving an analgesic can be distinguished from cats receiving a placebo up until the second day home (third day of treatment); after that, the cats are indistinguishable using behavioral criteria (unpublished observations). This suggests that 48 hours, and perhaps 72 or more hours, of analgesic treatment may be indicated, depending on the surgery or medical condition. Specific cases will be discussed in chapter 6.

## References


1. Hansen B, Hardie E. Prescription and use of analgesics in dogs and cats in a veterinary teaching hospital: 258 cases (1983–1989). J Am Vet Med Assoc 1993; 202:1485–94.
2. Dohoo SE, Dohoo IR. Postoperative use of analgesics in dogs and cats by Canadian veterinarians. Can Vet J 1996; 37:546–51.
3. Hubbell JAE, Muir WW. Evaluation of a survey of the diplomates of the American College of Laboratory Animal Medicine on use of analgesic agents in animals used in biomedical research. J Am Vet Med Assoc 1996; 209:918–21.
4. Benedetti C, Bonica JJ, Bellucci G. Pathophysiology and therapy of postoperative pain: a review. In: Benedetti C, Chapman CR, Moricca G, eds. Advances in pain research and therapy (vol 7). New York: Raven Press, 1984:373–407.
5. Bednarski RM. Anesthesia and pain control. Vet Clin of North Am: Small Animal Practice 1989; 19:1223–28.
6. Fraser RA, Hotz SB, Hurtig JB, Hodges SN, Moher D. The prevalence and impact of pain after day-care tubal ligation surgery. Pain 1989; 39:189–201.
7. Hardie EM, Hansen BD, Carroll GS. Behavior after ovariohysterectomy in the dog: what's normal? Appl Anim Behav 1997; 51:111–28.
8. Liles JH, Flecknell PA. The effects of surgical stimulus on the rat and the influence of analgesic treatment. Br Vet J 1993; 149:515.
9. Morton DB, Griffiths PHM. Guidelines on the recognition of pain, distress, and discomfort in experimental animals and an hypothesis for assessment. Vet Rec 1985; 116:431–36.
10. Reid J, Nolan AM. A comparison of the postoperative analgesic and sedative effects of flunixin and papaveretum in the dog. J Sm Animal Prac 1991; 32:603–8.
11. Day TK, Pepper WT, Tobias TA, Flynn MF, Clarke KM. Comparison of intra-articular and epidural morphine for analgesia following stifle arthrotomy in dogs. Vet Surg 1995; 24:522–30.
12. Crane SW. Perioperative analgesia: a surgeon's perspective. J Am Vet Med Assoc 1987; 191:1254–57.
13. Association of Veterinary Teachers and Research Workers. Guidelines for the recognition and assessment of pain in animals. Herts: Universities Federation for Animal Welfare, 1989.

14. Mroczek NS. Recognizing animal suffering and pain. Lab Animal 1992; 21:27–31.

15. Flecknell P. Advances in the assessment and alleviation of pain in laboratory and domestic animals. J Vet Anaesth 1994; 21: 98–105.

16. Smith JD, Allen SW, Quandt JE, Tackett RL. Indicators of postoperative pain in cats. Am J Vet Res 1996; 57:1674–78.

17. Popilskis S, Kohn DF, Laurent L, Danilo P. Efficacy of epidural morphine versus intravenous morphine for post-thoracotomy pain in dogs. J Vet Anaesth 1993; 20:21–25.

18. Hansen BD, Hardie EM, Carroll GS. Physiological measurements after ovariohysterectomy in dogs: what's normal? Appl Anim Behav 1997; 51:101–9.

19. Benson GJ, Wheaton LG, Thurmon JC, Tranquilli WJ, Olson WA, Davis CA. Postoperative catecholamine response to onychectomy in isoflurane-anesthetized cats. Vet Surg 1991; 20:222–25.

20. Thompson SE, Johnson JM. Analgesia in dogs after intercostal thoracotomy. Vet Surg 1991; 20:73–77.

21. Holton LL, Scott EM, Nolan AM, Reid J, Welsh E, Flaherty D. Comparison of three methods for assessment of pain in dogs. J Am Vet Med Assoc 1998; 212:61–66.

22. Conzemius MG, Hill CM, Sammarco JL, Perkowski SZ. Correlation between subjective and objective measures used to determine severity of postoperative pain in dogs. J Am Vet Med Assoc 1997; 210:1619–22.

23. Cousins MJ. Management of postoperative pain. In: Proceedings of the International Anesthesia Research Society, 60th Congress. Las Vegas: International Anesthesia Research Society, 1986: 32–39.

24. Kehlet H. Stress free anaesthesia and surgery. Acta Anaesth Scand 1979; 23:503–4.

25. Page GG. The medical necessity of adequate pain management. Pain Forum 1996; 5:227–33.

# Chapter 3 Treatment Strategies for Managing Pain

A comfortable environment, appropriate nursing care, and numerous and varied drug therapies contribute to patient well-being.

## Therapy

Veterinarians can use several strategies to make patients more comfortable. They can manipulate the environment to provide a safe and warm area for patients that are recovering from surgery or suffering from a critical illness. Appropriate nursing care can also provide significant comfort to the hospitalized animal. Practitioners can administer drugs to relieve anxiety and pain; several techniques for delivering drugs are addressed in this chapter. Additionally, various techniques of physical therapy or alternative therapy that may contribute to patient comfort will be covered.

## Environmental Therapy

Manipulating the patient's environment in various ways will help the veterinarian to manage the patient's pain. Although it often will not be practical, patients may be habituated to the hospital environment preoperatively. The surroundings of hospitalized patients should be as comfortable as possible. The environmental temperature, noise level, and cohabitating species of the wards should be controlled. For example, a recovery ward that is warmer and quieter than the regular wards may enhance patient comfort; a calm, slightly darkened room, with soft music (in contrast to a bright, well-lit room with lots of noise) can make the patient feel more comfortable. If space allows, cats may be more comfort-

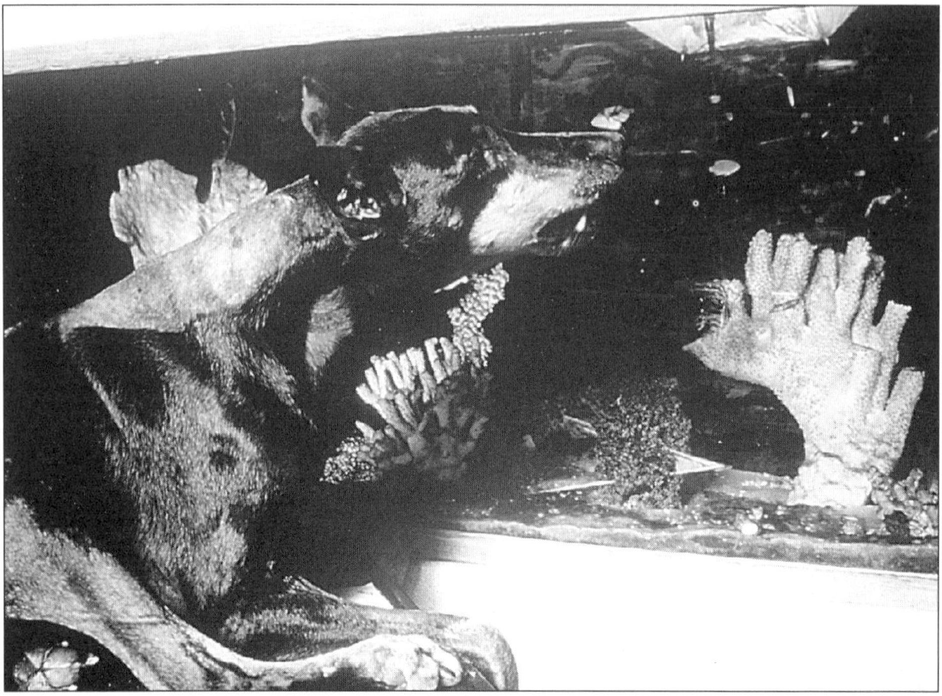

***Figure 3-1**. This Doberman watched fish when time allowed the attending clinician or student to take it into the waiting room. Ultimately, the owner brought in a TV for the dog to watch in the ward. (Photograph courtesy of Dr. Maryann Radlinsky.)*

able in wards without dogs. Many options exist for enhancing the environment of animals that will be hospitalized for an extended time. For example, in the case of a Doberman Pinscher recovering from surgery for stabilization of the cervical spine, the dog appeared to "enjoy" trips to the hospital's admitting area to watch tropical fish (see Figure 3-1). Based on this, the dog's owners provided a television in the ward to create a varied atmosphere, with the intent of decreasing the animal's level of boredom during the several months it was hospitalized. Such efforts may help to decrease the stress associated with a prolonged hospital stay.

With respect to anesthetic induction, each patient's care can be individualized in a number of inexpensive ways. The patient can be induced and recover in a warm, quiet, safe environment. For example, a hand-raised wallaby that had been raised in a purse was presented for anesthesia. The wallaby would have been stressed by attempts to remove it from the purse; it was

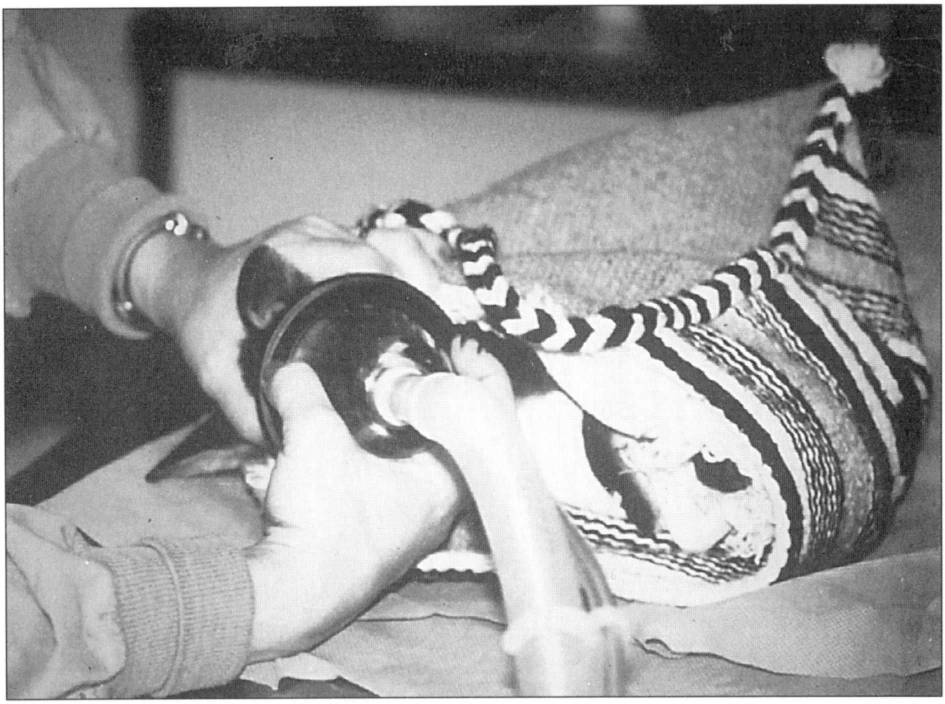

***Figure 3-2**. Both gentle handling and a quiet, calm anesthetic induction can reduce perioperative stress, as is illustrated for this hand-raised wallaby.*
***Figure 3-2 A.** The wallaby was content to be mask-induced if allowed to stay in the purse in which it was raised.*

quite content to be mask-induced with isoflurane while it remained in the purse (see Figure 3-2 A). It was easy to remove the wallaby from the purse after anesthetic induction (see Figure 3-2 B).

Patients should be as comfortable as possible after surgery. A quick checklist of ways to facilitate this may be helpful:

- Express the bladder.
- Lubricate the eyes.
- Position the animal so that pressure is not placed on surgical sites, using adequate padding to prevent decubital ulcers.
- Support the head and limbs with pillows or rolled towels when appropriate.
- Turn patients every 2 to 3 hours if they are unable to reposition themselves.
- Place proper bandages (not too tight) and appropriately stabilize fractures.

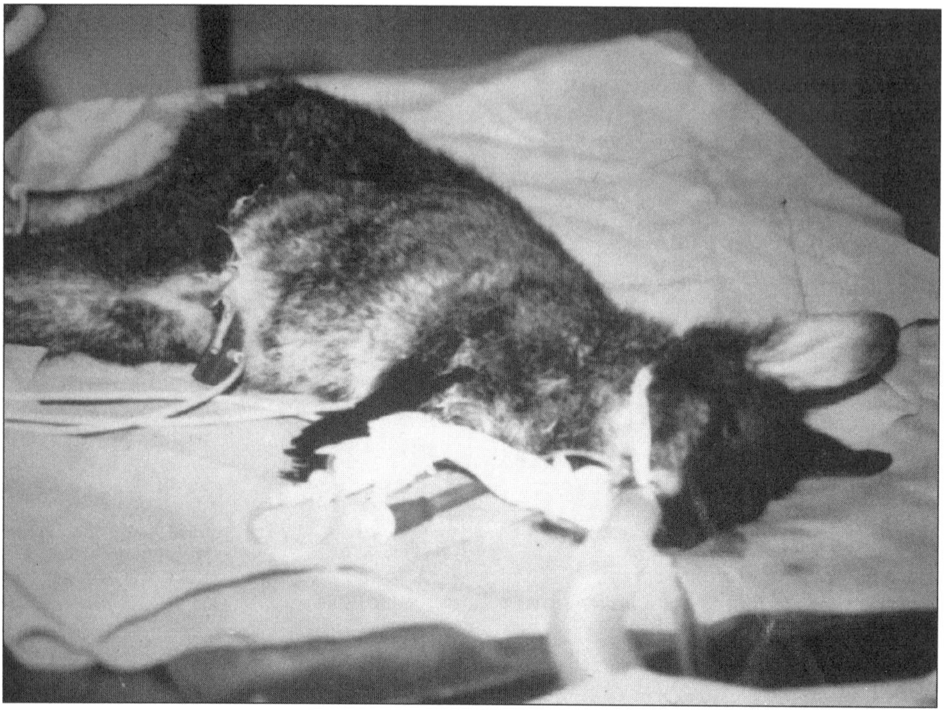

*Figure 3-2 B. Once induced, the wallaby was removed from the purse; handling stress was minimized.*

- Remove any dried blood or irritating soap from the skin.
- Use plastic sheets with absorbent liners to keep patients dry.

## Drug Therapy

Many of the other treatments for pain and discomfort involve drug therapy. Analgesics seem to be the only medications that are routinely withheld when there is a question about their need. Tranquilization may relieve anxiety and enhance patient cooperation, but tranquilization does not relieve pain. Tranquilizers (acepromazine, diazepam) should not be used alone in painful animals. Only after adequate analgesia has been provided is it appropriate to tranquilize a patient (if indicated). More importantly, it is generally more difficult to assess pain in a heavily tranquilized or sedated animal. A veterinarian may mistake an outwardly sedate animal for a pain-free animal. Generally, tranquilizers are administered preoperatively to relieve anxiety and postoperatively to combat dysphoria (e.g., restlessness) or emergence delirium. If procedures are invasive, administering an analgesic preoperatively will provide preemptive analgesia (discussed later in this chapter). It may be necessary to adjust the dose of the analgesic postoperatively, depending on how long the administered analgesic is effective and how well the patient is recovering from the anesthesia. Administration of a postoperative tranquilizer may be considered if adequate analgesia has been assured. Tranquilizing a patient without analgesia would be appropriate for noninvasive procedures, such as radiography or endoscopy without biopsy, which do not result in postoperative pain.

## Tranquilization and Sedation

Tranquilization and sedation in small animal medicine are restricted to administering tranquilizers (e.g., acepromazine, diazepam) and $\alpha_2$-agonists (e.g., xylazine, medetomidine). Clinically, acepromazine, an $\alpha$-antagonist, may cause profound hypotension and should be used cautiously in animals with volume depletion. Other reported side effects of acepromazine include a lowered seizure threshold and decreased platelet aggregation. The effects of acepromazine may last longer in old or ill patients and in patients with hepatic disease; there are no specific antagonists for acepromazine. When acepromazine is indicated for tranquilization in young, healthy, normotensive animals with no contraindications to the drug, practitioners should administer it (0.05 mg/kg [not to exceed 1 mg], IM or SC) (see Figure 3-3). In geriatric patients or in patients in which hemorrhage or hypotension during surgery is anticipated, wait to administer acepromazine (0.05 mg/kg [not to exceed 1 mg], IV titrated to effect) until during or after recovery, and then only if the patient is dysphoric or excited.

Diazepam, a benzodiazepine derivative, is an unreliable tranquilizer when used alone in small animal medicine. Diazepam may cause disinhibition of learned behavior and may induce excitement. Diazepam in very young, very old, or very ill animals provides more reliable sedation than in healthy middle-aged animals. Generally, administer diazepam (0.2 mg/kg, IV) after administration of an opioid. Few cardiopulmonary effects are associated with administering diazepam. Additionally,

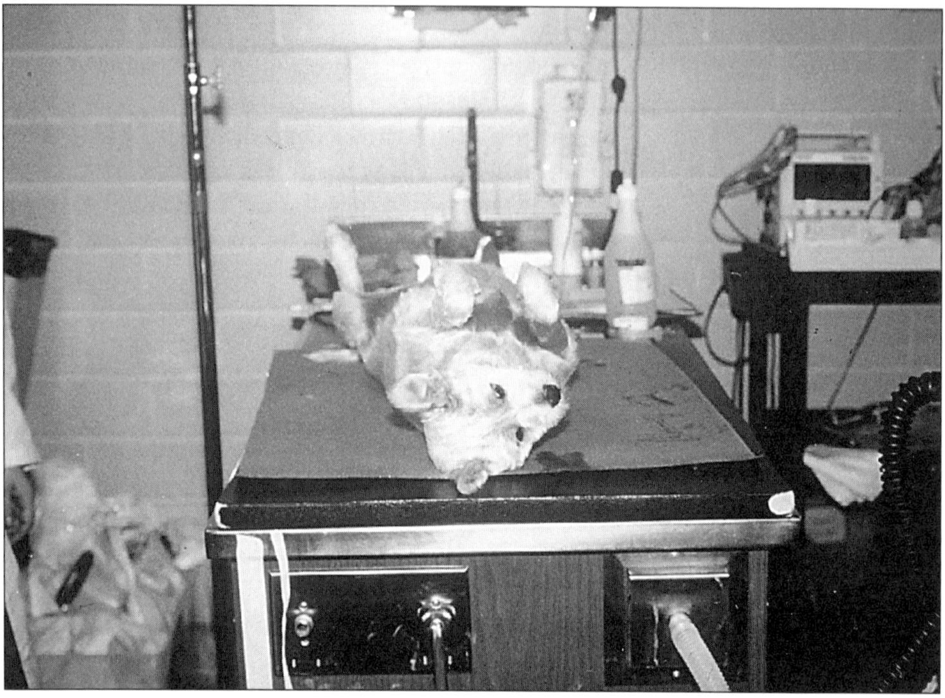

***Figure 3-3**. A relaxed patient after receiving acepromazine prior to surgery (an attendant is close by).*

flumazenil (0.011 to 0.022 mg/kg, IV[1] titrated to effect) is a specific antagonist for diazepam.

Xylazine and medetomidine are $\alpha_2$-agonists that cause dose-dependent sedation and cardiopulmonary depression, and profound analgesia. These drugs provide analgesia through a non-opioid system and are not controlled (i.e., scheduled). Both are excellent drugs for restraint, but should be used with caution when administering them for perioperative analgesia, particularly in critical or injured animals. When an $\alpha_2$-agonist is used as an anesthetic adjunct in young, healthy animals undergoing elective procedures, substantial analgesia may be provided.[2] Two caveats: The sedation caused by these drugs outlasts the analgesia, and cardiopulmonary depression may be profound.

Very low doses of $\alpha_2$-agonists may profoundly increase analgesia and sedation when administered with an opioid. Alpha$_2$-agonists and opioids have been shown to have a synergistic effect for analgesia in some models. Xylazine is the classic $\alpha_2$-agonist; medetomidine is a newer member of the group and for some sick and injured animals may offer fewer systemic side effects than xylazine.[2] However, postoperative doses and duration of medetomidine are not well established and should be used cautiously to avoid cardiovascular depression. Additionally, postsurgical doses to be used concurrently with opioids are not well established.[3]

Alpha$_2$-antagonists (e.g., yohimbine, atipamezole, tolazoline) will antagonize the effects of the $\alpha_2$-agonist drugs. Alpha$_2$-antagonists produce some side effects; practitioners should use them with caution, particularly in painful animals. Antagonism of $\alpha_2$-agonists has been associated with deaths in cattle[4] and sheep,[5] and with an increased concentration of stress-related hormones and metabolites in horses.[6] It may be prudent to obtain the desired dose of antagonist and titrate it intravenously to effect.

**Analgesia**

Current anesthetic practices rely on induction agents such as propofol and thiopental, which offer speedy recoveries but little analgesia, and inhalation agents such as isoflurane or sevoflurane that are associated with rapid recoveries. In people, patients that receive isoflurane need more postoperative analgesics than patients that receive halothane or enflurane;[7] clinically, the same appears to be true for animals. A speedy recovery may be an advantage for outpatient surgeries, but may leave a patient without residual analgesia.

Historically in small animal medicine, veterinarians have used only opioid analgesics in the immediate perioperative period. Alpha$_2$-agonists, local anesthetics, and nonsteroidal anti-inflammatory drugs (NSAIDs) are used in addition to opioids in large animal medicine. Local anesthetics and NSAIDs are gaining favor in small animal anesthesia; residual (postoperative) effects of $\alpha_2$-agonists may provide analgesia. Ketamine, a dissociative anesthetic, has also been used for somatic pain. Specific analgesic drugs are discussed in chapter 4.

If analgesics are to be administered, when is the best time? It is sensible to provide an agent that will offer intraoperative as well as postoperative analgesia. "Preemptive" analgesia (administering an analgesic before stimulating nociception) is based on the concept that analgesia administered before the noxious stimulus outlasts the analgesic's duration of action in the body.[8] For postoperative analgesia to be most effective, the process of nociception should be inhibited with analgesics prior to initiation of the painful stimulus.[2,9,10] Noxious afferent signals during surgery contribute to central nervous system sensitization and increased postoperative pain.[11] For example, patients that received lumbar epidural administration of fentanyl 15 minutes before surgical incision had significantly lower pain scores and morphine requirements postoperatively than patients that received lumbar epidural administration of fentanyl 15 minutes after incision.[11]

Central sensitization and *wind-up* (the hyperexcitable state resulting from an afferent volley of nociceptive impulses) appear to be dependent on the activation of N-methyl-D-aspartic acid (NMDA) receptors; NMDA receptor antagonists may prevent or reverse central sensitization.[10] C-fiber excitatory amino acids and neuropeptides seemingly facilitate plasticity of dorsal horn spinal cord neurons initiated by noxious stimulation.[10] Intracellular second messengers, rather than the shorter postsynaptic actions of C-fiber excitatory amino acids and neuropeptides, may initiate prolonged nociceptive changes in neural function after NMDA receptors have been activated.[10]

Although opioid analgesics diminish wind-up, local anesthetics that block afferent and efferent pathways are more effective in preventing wind-up. There is also evidence that administering preemptive NMDA receptor antagonists (e.g., ketamine) decreases wound hyperalgesia.[8]

Another advantage of administering an opioid or local anesthetic preoperatively is that less inhalant is required intraoperatively. The disadvantage to preoperative administration, depending on the analgesic used and the surgical time, is that doing so will not provide analgesia for very long into the postoperative period. So, postoperative analgesia may be insufficient if drugs are not repeated.

*Therapeutic Techniques (Drug-Delivery Options)*

Drug-delivery systems for analgesics are varied and, to a certain extent, depend on the type of drug being administered. For example, the most commonly used technique for administering opioids is systemically on a schedule (e.g., IV every 4 hours); however, opioids may also be administered using regional techniques (e.g., epidurally). Conversely, local anesthetics are generally applied with regional techniques (e.g., epidurally), but may be administered IV by infusion in dogs.

With respect to scheduled systemic administration, analgesics may be delivered orally or by injection (IM, SC, IV). Generally, in conscious animals, it is preferable to administer them by IV (if an IV catheter is available) in order to avoid painful IM injections. When analgesics are administered on a schedule, the treatment goal is to maintain blood levels in a therapeutic range. With most analgesics, comparative pharmacokinetic data are not available for all veterinary species; the predicted duration of activity is based on clinical response or duration of activity in other species. Invariably, in some treatment intervals, the concentration of the analgesic will not reach or will exceed therapeutic concentrations. It is more difficult to control a patient's pain if the patient is allowed to experience pain before treatment, which suggests that administering analgesics as needed (e.g., PRN) is less desirable than using scheduled therapy. Methods are being developed that will allow for encapsulation of analgesic microcrystals with lecithin to prolong analgesic delivery (time-released delivery).[12] Other methods of drug delivery, including continuous infusion and transdermal administration (see Figure 3-4 A), may provide more constant blood levels.

Several drugs (e.g., morphine, fentanyl) may be administered intravenously by constant rate infusion (CRI). CRI is particularly beneficial for patients whose pain cannot be controlled with intermittent injections. For CRI administration, drugs may be delivered by syringe pump or added to a compatible fluid and administered over an appropriate time. When a beginning infusion rate is known and when the drug's duration of action is relatively brief (e.g., fentanyl), a

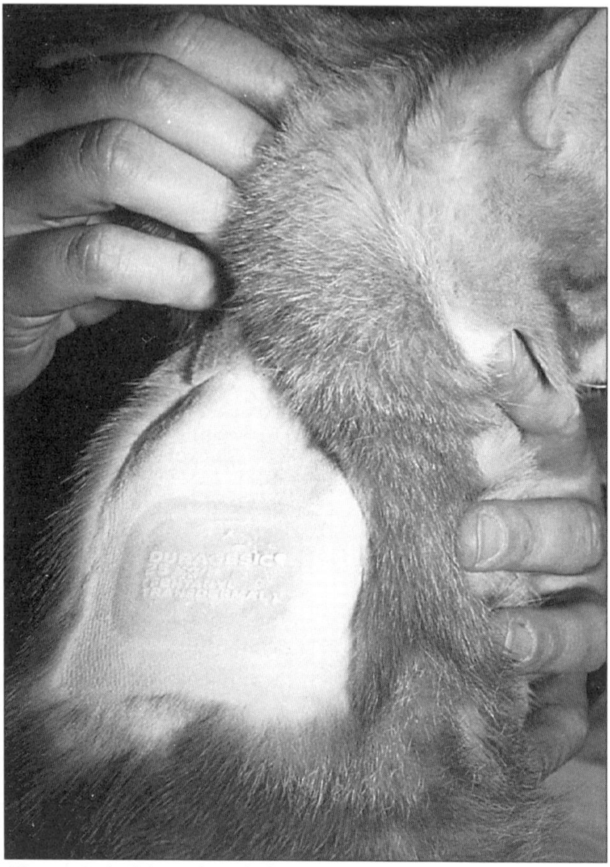

***Figure 3-4**. This series of photographs illustrates appropriate placement of a transdermal fentanyl patch in a domestic short-haired cat.*
***Figure 3-4 A.** The transdermal fentanyl patch in place.*

loading dose is administered, an infusion begun, and the dose adjusted based on clinical response. For drugs that have a longer duration of action (e.g., morphine), the infusion dose is established by first determining a loading dose (i.e., administering small incremental doses every few minutes until the desired clinical effect is achieved) and then administering that dose over the drug's anticipated duration of action. For specific examples of administering drugs by CRI, see the individual drugs described in chapter 4.

To administer a drug transdermally, the hair over the lateral thorax or dorsal cervical region (the axillary area in cats is also a good location) should be clipped without damaging the skin (i.e., avoid "clipper burns")

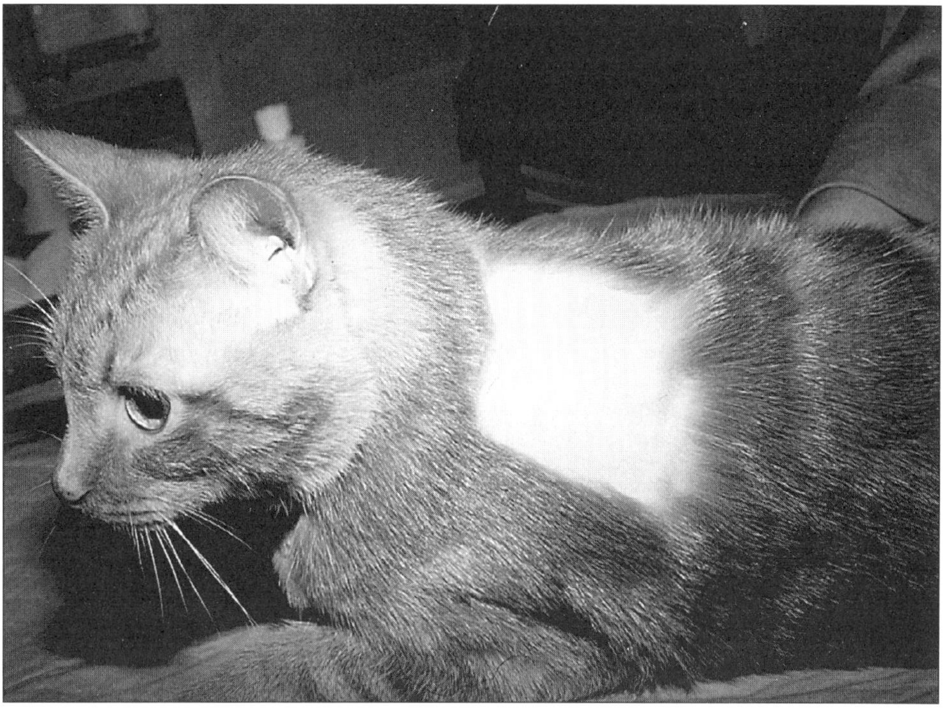

***Figure 3-4B.*** *The hair is clipped over the dorsal cervical region for the placement of a fentanyl transdermal patch. The site should not be scrubbed.*

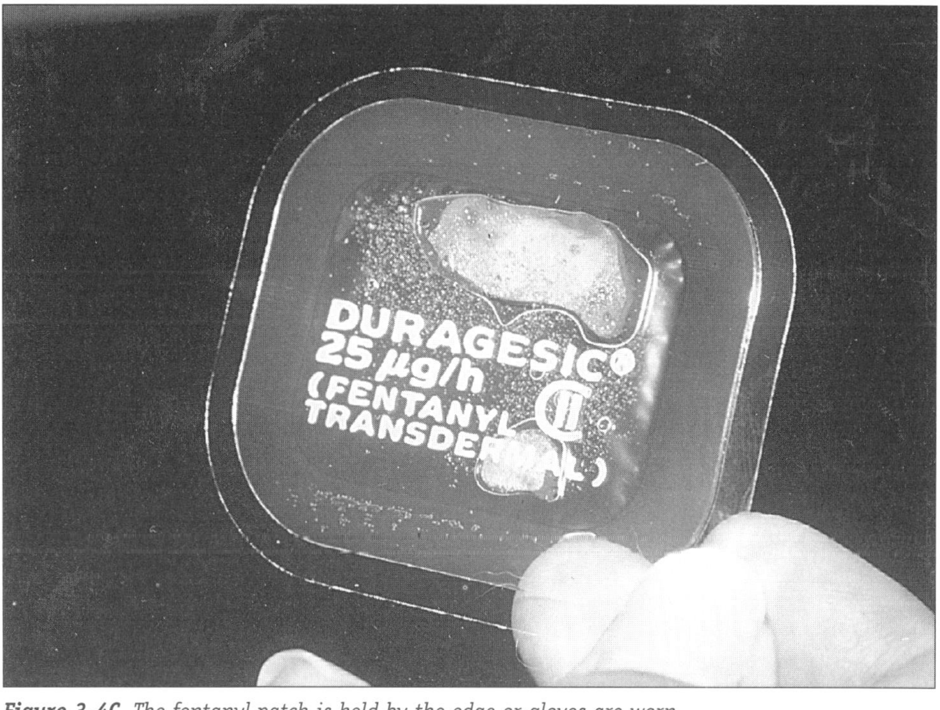


***Figure 3-4C.*** *The fentanyl patch is held by the edge or gloves are worn.*

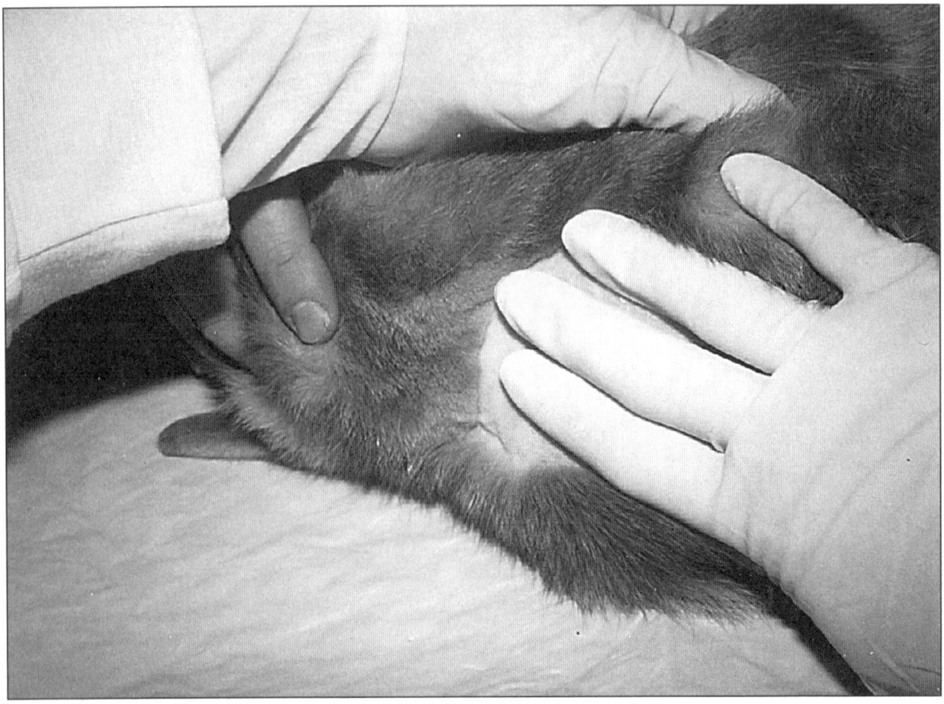

***Figure 3-4D***. *The fentanyl patch is held in place for 2 minutes.*

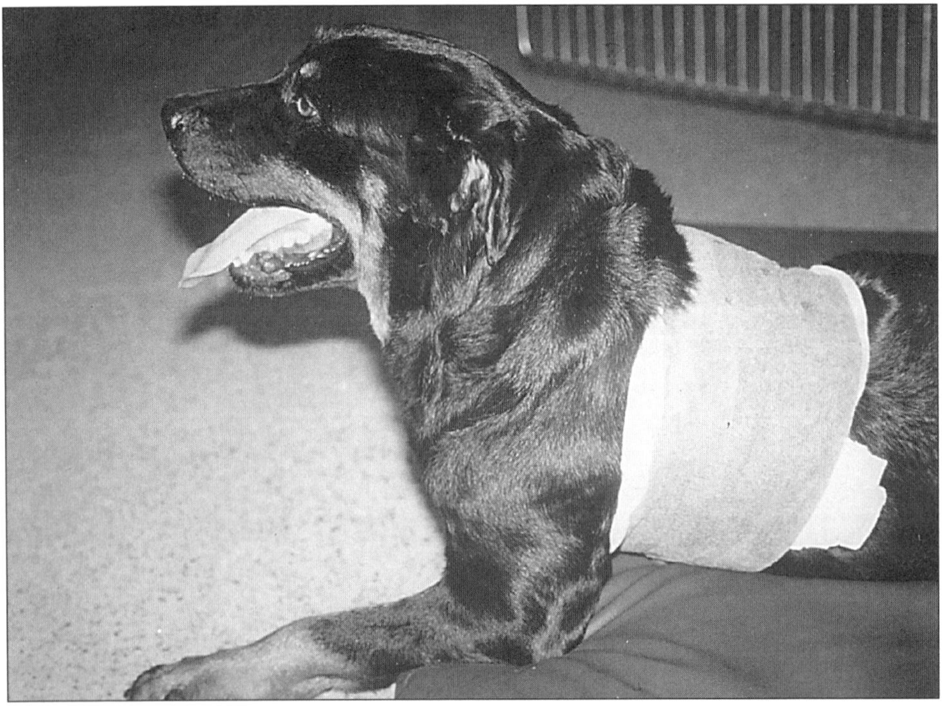

***Figure 3-5***. *A lightly bandaged fentanyl patch on a dog that has undergone forelimb amputation. (Photograph courtesy of Ms. Dana Heath.)*

(see Figure 3-4 B). The site should not be cleaned with alcohol or surgical scrub. The patch should be handled by the edge or gloves should be worn to avoid contact with the membrane (see Figure 3-4 C). It is important to hold the patch in place for 2 minutes (see Figure 3-4 D). In dogs, the site should be bandaged (see Figure 3-5); in cats, covering the patch may not be necessary. Tissue adhesive should not be used to increase the adhesiveness of the patch to the skin, since the glue will interfere with the membrane and alter absorption. The location of the patch should be carefully considered so that during surgery, the patch and the skin below it will not be exposed to increased heat (i.e., avoid direct contact with a warm-water circulating blanket). Fever may also increase absorption of fentanyl from a patch. When removing a patch, wear gloves, fold the patch on itself, and flush it down a toilet in the presence of a witness.

Veterinarians are increasingly implementing local anesthetic and local analgesic techniques in small animal medicine, using local anesthetics and opioids. *Local anesthesia* refers to both afferent and efferent blockade; *local analgesia* refers to a decrease or loss of only a sensory component. Local anesthesia has been shown to decrease the intensity of postoperative pain beyond the expected duration of the local anesthetic.[9] As discussed earlier, this probably occurs through the suppression of the nerve's hyperexcitable state, which may be responsible for maintaining a degree of postoperative pain.[9] Local anesthetics are not very efficacious in infected wounds.

Although veterinarians have long accepted the efficacy of opioids in the epidural space and spinal fluid, new evidence suggests that peripheral opioid receptors also contribute to analgesia. Most veterinarians have little clinical experience with peripheral opioid receptors in veterinary patients since this area of research is relatively new. In people, intra-articular morphine in the stifle has been effective, but not other modes of administering peripheral opioids (e.g., ankle and axillary, intraperitoneal and interpleural).[13] In dogs, intra-articular[14,15] but not interpleural[16] morphine has been proven to be efficacious. In dogs, intra-articular morphine (0.1 mg/kg diluted in 1 ml of saline/10 kg of body weight) was compared to epidural morphine (0.1 mg/kg diluted in 1 ml of saline/5 kg of body weight). Intra-articular morphine provided analgesia equivalent to that which epidural morphine offered. Both groups had lower pain scores than groups treated with saline.[14] Also, in dogs, intra-articular morphine (0.1 mg/kg diluted with saline to 0.5 ml/kg of body weight) and intra-articular bupivacaine (0.5% at 0.5 ml/kg) provided better analgesia than saline in stifle surgery, with bupivacaine showing the greatest effect.[15] Morphine (1.0 mg/kg, IM or 1.0 mg/kg, interpleurally) was compared to interpleural bupivacaine (0.5%, 1.5 mg/kg) in dogs. Compared to IM administration of morphine, interpleural morphine did not appear to provide any advantages with respect to pulmonary function or analgesia.[16] Interpleural bupivacaine produced the fewest blood gas abnormalities. Pain scores did not differ.[16]

Administering anesthetics and analgesics epidurally is becoming popular for perioperative analgesia (Appendix A describes this technique). Many types of drugs have been administered in the epidural space (e.g., local anesthetics, opioids, $\alpha_2$-agonists, ketamine); in small animal medicine, the preferred drugs are generally local anesthetics or opioids. Potential complications from administering any drug epidurally include infection, hemorrhage, and failure to produce analgesia or anesthesia. Hypovolemia is a contraindication for administering local anesthetics epidurally, since blocking the sympathetic system will promote hypotension. To avoid the risk of neurotoxicity, it is best to use preservative-free drugs when administering drugs epidurally. Administering phenol and formaldehyde (preservatives) epidurally is associated with adverse reactions, including both central nervous system and local epidural tissue toxicity.[17] Methylparaben, as a preservative, is associated with minimal risk.[18] It is prudent for veterinarians to avoid administering any substance epidurally that would cause neural damage if it were administered intrathecally, since inadvertent spinal administration may occur. It is extremely important to avoid contamination; using single-dose vials reduces the risk of introducing infection from a contaminated drug.[18]

Administering different classes of drugs epidurally offers various benefits and disadvantages. If the veterinarian expects the patient to be able to ambulate immediately postoperatively, epidural opioids offer analgesia without motor dysfunction. With respect to local anesthetic epidurals, bupivacaine appears to attenuate or block sensory nerves with less impairment of motor function than does lidocaine. Regarding cardiac function, administering local anesthetics can decrease heart rate, cardiac output, and blood pressure; postural hypotension may occur. Administering opioids epidurally usually does not change the patient's heart rate, but may minimally decrease heart rate; epidural opioids at therapeutic doses generally do not decrease cardiac output or blood pressure; the vasoconstrictor response remains intact. Administering local anesthetics at appropriate doses epidurally usually does not impair the respiratory system unless the local anesthetic migrates cranially; avoid a head-down tilt to the surgery table. Administering opioids epidurally may cause early respiratory depression due to systemic absorption or late (6- to 24-hour) respiratory depression due to opioid migration to the brain, but this is extremely uncommon in dogs and cats. The respiratory depression may be treated with naloxone. Administering anesthetics locally results in mild or no sedation, although central nervous system toxicity may occur if a large dose of a local anesthetic is administered. Administering opioids epidurally may result in sedation; infrequently, it causes nausea, vomiting, and pruritus. With either local anesthetics or opioids, retention of urine may occur.

What are the indications for administering local anesthetics or opioids for analgesia spinally or epidurally? Epidurals are useful for intraoperative analgesia in high-risk patients (to decrease the requirements for other depressants), for perioperative analgesia (particularly if surgery will be delayed), for caudal anesthesia or analgesia (perineum, hindlimbs, tail, abdomen), and depending on the agent chosen, for some thoracotomies and forelimb amputations. Epidural catheters may be employed in patients that will require repeated doses of the selected drug (e.g., a patient with a pelvic fracture awaiting stabilization).

It may be necessary to adjust the epidural dosage if the patient has certain preexisting conditions. Obesity, distension of epidural veins, space-occupying lesions in the spinal canal, and increased CSF volume (increased volume of the dural sac) decrease the size of the epidural space; the volume and dose of the drug should be decreased to limit spread of the drug craniad. The dose should also be decreased if the patient is pregnant, since increased intra-abdominal pressure enhances cranial migration. Elderly patients have progressively occluded intervertebral foramina and thus a smaller epidural space. If cerebrospinal fluid is encountered while performing the epidural, the dose of the local anesthetic should be decreased by approximately half; generally, the dose of the opioid is not decreased if cerebrospinal fluid is encountered.

Perhaps the least technical and easiest local anesthetic techniques to perform are those involving local infiltration of drugs. These may be performed as line blocks, splash blocks (bathing the affected area), nerve root injections, or joint infusions. These techniques are generally reserved for local anesthetics, although opioids have proven effective in joint infusions. Infiltration techniques are simple to perform because the involved area is readily available. As a general rule, do not exceed the maximum dose of local anesthetic that should be used for a given patient (see recommendations for specific drugs in chapter 4); dilute the dose if a greater volume is required. Incisional pain may be controlled with line blocks. Line blocks have been used extensively in food animal medicine and surgery; many small animal practitioners have implemented line blocks for Cesarean sections in order to reduce the need for injectable and inhalant anesthetics. With longer-acting local anesthetics, line blocks may control incisional pain for up to 8 hours. Similarly, ring blocks, around a digit or tail, are effective; clinically, local anesthetic ring blocks at the level of the carpus for an onychectomy appear effective for postoperative analgesia in cats (Hellyer, personal communication). Splash blocks may be used to supplement analgesia in particularly painful surgical procedures. Splash blocks are routinely used for ear ablations and onychectomies (see Case Study No. 3 in chapter 6). Recent studies[19,20] have been unable to demonstrate a measurable advantage over traditional methods of analgesia in these two procedures, but clinically, patients appear to benefit from these techniques; further evaluation with more sensitive tests for analgesia is needed before these techniques are abandoned. In order for a splash block to be effective, sufficient contact time for the particular agent must be allowed (e.g., about 20 minutes of contact time for bupivacaine; in general, the longer-acting the local anesthetic agent, the longer the onset time). When a forelimb or hindlimb is amputated, the nerve stumps may be injected directly with a local anesthetic to supplement analgesia.

A brachial plexus block (see Appendix A) may be used for forelimb amputations instead of injecting the nerve stump. Although this is technically more difficult to perform, blocking the brachial plexus before surgery allows the full advantage of preemptive analgesia from local anesthetics. Brachial plexus anesthesia blocks the region from the foot up to the elbow (radial, median, ulnar, musculocutaneous, axillary nerves).

Pain associated with thoracotomy can be managed with intercostal neural blockade, interpleural analgesia, and systemic or selected epidural opioids. Respiratory depression from potent opioids may be a concern for some thoracotomy patients, but pain-free patients usually ventilate better than painful patients; thoracotomy patients generally tolerate opioids well. Normally, local anesthetic techniques for treating thoracotomy pain provide analgesia without respiratory depression. During an intercostal nerve block, the intercostal nerves are directly blocked. The intercostal nerves that supply the incision site, two nerves cranial and two nerves caudal to the thoracotomy incision are selectively blocked (see Figures 3-6 A to 3-6 C). Due to the overlap of innervation, three consecutive intercostal nerves must be blocked. To accomplish an intercostal block, the injection is made just caudal to each rib near the intervertebral foramen. Potential complica-

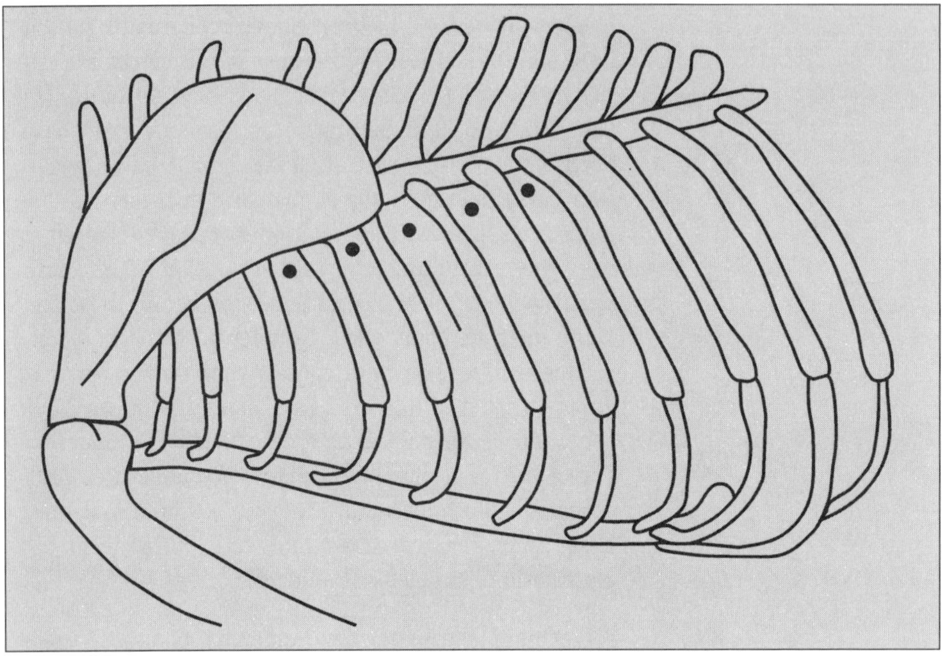

***Figure 3-6***. *The line drawing of a cat and photographs of a dog indicate proper application of an intercostal nerve block technique for thoracotomy incision or placement of a thoracic drain.*
***Figure 3-6 A***. *For an intercostal nerve block, two nerves in front and two nerves behind the incision site are blocked.*

tions include respiratory failure due to motor blockade, pneumothorax, and inadvertent overdosage of the local anesthetic. However, this procedure has been used for many years, and is considered to be very safe.

Interpleural analgesia is an alternative or supplement to intercostal neural blockade for post-thoracotomy pain. Interpleural analgesia offers prolonged analgesia without multiple injections.[16,21] Local anesthetic (bupivacaine) is diluted with saline and instilled through a thoracic drain. The patient is positioned with the operative site down for 15 to 20 minutes. If the thoracic drain is left in place, additional bupivacaine can be administered postoperatively (every 6 hours). In conscious patients that are sleeping, it is important to awaken them before instilling bupivacaine into the thorax; administering a cold and potentially stingy substance into the thorax of a sleeping animal has precipitated arrhythmias, presumably from catecholamine release. Potential complications associated with interpleural analgesia include pneumothorax and

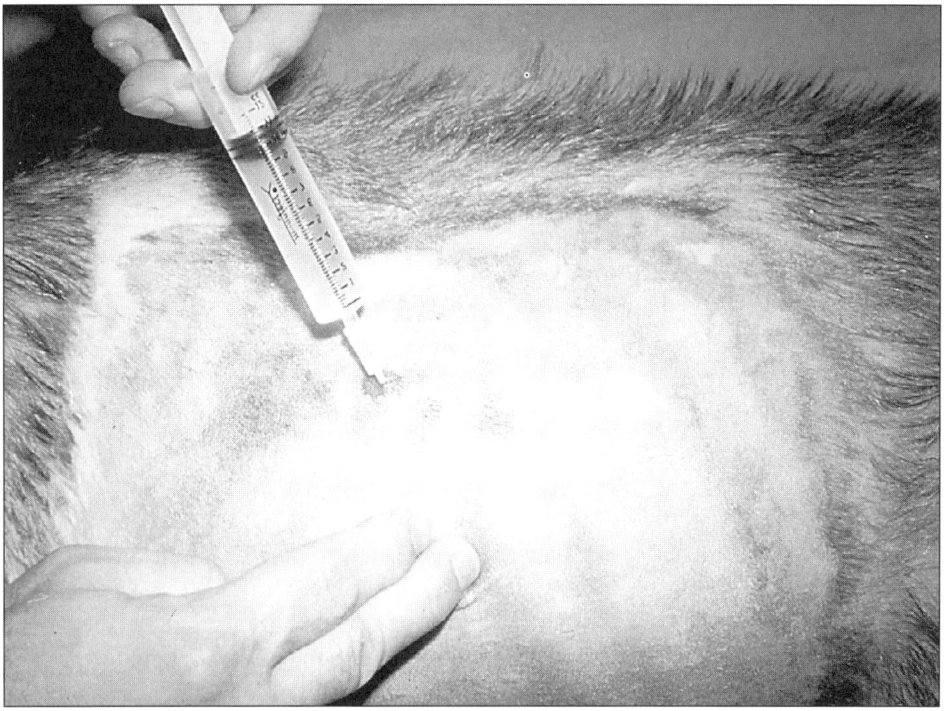

***Figure 3-6 B.*** *The intercostal nerves are blocked for a thoracic drain in this dog. (Photograph courtesy of Dr. Sandee Hartsfield.)*

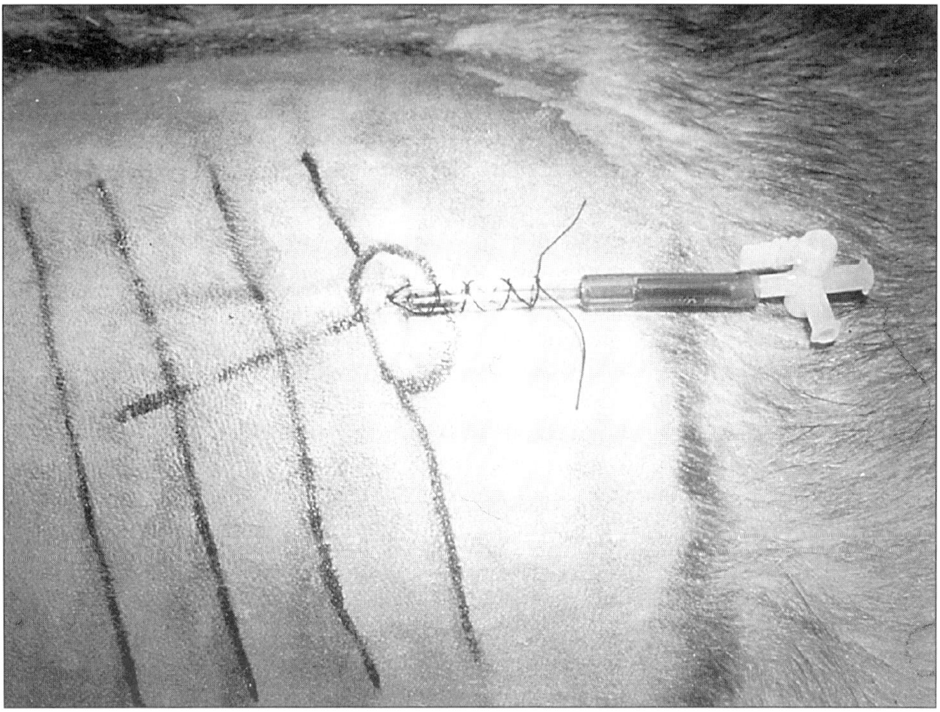

***Figure 3-6 C.*** *The thoracic drain was successfully placed with sedation and intercostal nerve blocks. (Photograph courtesy of Dr. Sandee Hartsfield.)*

inadvertent overdosage of local anesthetic. Various theoretical concerns regarding the involvement of multiple neural structures have not proved to be clinically relevant. Practitioners should avoid administering local anesthetics interpleurally in patients with an open pericardium. Intercostal and interpleural blocks may be combined if the maximum dose of local anesthetic is not exceeded (see chapter 4 for dosage guidelines).

## Physical Therapy

Veterinarians are using massage, exercise (active and passive), and hydrotherapy to help patients with severe tissue injury to recover. The benefits of using these techniques are early return of function, maintaining range of motion, and decreased fibrosis and atrophy of muscle.[22] Physical therapy may improve an animal's mental status and decrease hospitalization time.[22] Massage (stroking, kneading, friction) increases blood flow and lymph flow; it is important not to exceed an individual's tolerance for pain.[22] Exercise strengthens, maintains, and improves function. Passive exercise (flexion, extension of joints through normal range of motion) prevents stiffness.[22] Active exercise requires voluntary motor control, but may be assisted.[22] Hydrotherapy increases circulation and may provide some analgesia.[22] Individuals seem to respond well to appropriate intervention.

## Alternative Therapy

Veterinarians are using acupuncture, magnetic therapy, and holistic herb therapy for patients that have not responded to conventional therapy. Clients and some veterinarians seek alternative therapy when conventional therapy fails to provide relief for veterinary patients.[23]

Acupuncture has been used effectively to control postoperative pain and to provide surgical analgesia, although it is not without limitations (e.g., inadequate analgesia, lack of restraint, lack of knowledge regarding points).[24] Acupuncture appears to be particularly beneficial for chronic pain syndromes.[25] The American Veterinary Medical Association considers acupuncture and acutherapy to be valid modalities, but with a potential for abuse.[26] Pet owners and veterinarians should choose an acupuncturist carefully; the International Veterinary Acupuncture Society offers a course to teach and certify veterinarians in acupuncture techniques.[25] Using veterinary acupuncture has been reviewed,[27,28] and controlled studies are being conducted.[29,30]

There are few controlled studies that have examined the outcome of chiropractic therapy, homeopathy, botanical medicine, nutraceutical medicine, and holistic medicine. The American Veterinary Medical Association has published guidelines for alternative and complementary veterinary care;[31] veterinarians should examine these guidelines before undertaking alternative therapies. As alternative therapies are examined in controlled studies, it is perhaps important to keep an open mind regarding such treatments when conventional medicine fails to provide relief.

## References


1. Muir WW, Hubbell JAE. Handbook of Veterinary Anesthesia. St. Louis: CV Mosby Co, 1989.
2. Hansen BD. Analgesic therapy. Compendium Continuing Educ Practicing Vet 1994; 16:868–75.
3. Hellyer PW, Gaynor JS. Acute postsurgical pain in dogs and cats. Compendium Continuing Educ Practicing Vet 1998; 20:140–53.
4. Kitzman JV, Booth NH, Hatch RC, Wallner B. Antagonism of xylazine sedation by 4-aminopyridine and yohimbine in cattle. Am J Vet Res 1982; 43:2165–69.
5. Hsu WH, Schaffer DD, Hanson CE. Effects of tolazoline and yohimbine on xylazine-induced central nervous system depression, bradycardia, and tachypnea in sheep. J Am Vet Med Assoc 1987; 190:423–26.
6. Carroll GL, Matthews NS, Hartsfield SM, Slater MS, Champney TH, Erickson SW. The effect of detomidine and its antagonism with tolazoline on stress-related hormones, metabolites, physiologic responses, and behavior in awake ponies. Vet Surg 1997; 26:69–77.
7. Tracey JA, Holland AJC, Unger L. Morbidity in minor gynaecological surgery: a comparison of halothane, enflurane and isoflurane. Br J Anaesth 1982; 54:1213–15.
8. Tverskoy M, Oz Y, Isakson A, Finger J, Bradley EL, Kissin I. Preemptive effect of fentanyl and ketamine on postoperative pain and wound hyperalgesia. Anesth Analg 1994; 78:205–9.
9. Tverskoy M, Cozacov C, Ayache M, Bradley EL, Kissin I. Postoperative pain after inguinal herniorrhaphy with different types of anesthesia. Anesth Analg 1990; 70:29–35.
10. Katz J, Kavanagh BP, Sandler AN, et al. Preemptive analgesia. Anesthesiology 1992; 77:439–46.
11. Kavanagh BP, Katz J, Sandler AN. Pain control after thoracic surgery. Anesthesiology 1994; 81:737–59.
12. Boedeker BH, Lojeski EW, Kline MD, Haynes DH. Ultra-long-duration local anesthesia produced by injection of lecithin-coated tetracaine microcrystals. J Clin Pharm 1994; 34:699–702.

13. Stein C. The control of pain in peripheral tissue by opioids. N Engl J Med 1995; 332:1685–90.

14. Day TK, Pepper WT, Tobias TA, Flynn MF, Clarke KM. Comparison of intra-articular and epidural morphine for analgesia following stifle arthotomy in dogs. Vet Surg 1995; 24:522–30.

15. Sammarco JL, Conzemius MG, Perkowski SZ, Weinstein MJ, Gregor TP, Smith GK. Postoperative analgesia for stifle surgery: A comparison of intra-articular bupivacaine, morphine, or saline. Vet Surg 1996; 25:59–69.

16. Stobie D, Caywood DD, Rozanski EA, et al. Evaluation of pulmonary function and analgesia in dogs after intercostal thoracotomy and use of morphine administered intramuscularly or intrapleurally and bupivacaine administered intrapleurally. Am J Vet Res 1995; 56:1098–1109.

17. DuPen SL, Ramsey D, Chin S. Chronic epidural morphine and preservative-induced injury. Anesthesiology 1987; 67:987–88.

18. Pascoe P. Advantages and guidelines for using epidural drugs for analgesia. Vet Clin No Amer Sm Anim Prac 1992; 22:421–23.

19. Buback JL, Boothe HW, Carroll GL, Green RW. Comparison of three methods for relief of pain after ear canal ablation in dogs. Vet Surg 1996; 25:380–85.

20. Winkler KP, Greenfield CL, Benson GJ. The effect of wound irrigation with bupivacaine on postoperative analgesia of the feline onychectomy patient. J Am An Hosp Assoc 1997; 33: 346–52.

21. Robinson EP. Perioperative and postoperative pain control in the dog and cat. In: Animal pain and its control. Proceedings 226 in conjunction with the Chapter of Anaesthetics & Intensive Care of the Australian College of Veterinary Scientists. Sydney: Post Graduate Committee in Veterinary Science University of Sydney, 1994:423–39.

22. Sikes R. Postoperative management of the neurosurgical patient. Problems in Veterinary Medicine. Philadelphia: J. B. Lippincott Company, 1989; 1:467–77.

23. Gorman C. St. Bernard's Wort. Time 1997 Nov 3:93–94.

24. Klide AM. Acupuncture-produced surgical analgesia. Problems in Veterinary Medicine. Philadelphia: J. B. Lippincott Company 1992; 4:200–6.

25. Smith C. Acupuncture: an ancient treatment modality under scientific scrutiny. J Am Vet Med Assoc 1992; 201:1321–25.

26. Schoen AM. Acupuncture: through the eye of a needle. Veterinary Forum 1991; 8:24.

27. Clifford DH, Lee MO, Lee DC. The relationship between acupuncture and drugs: a review. Compendium Continuing Educ Practicing Vet 1980; 2:746–52.

28. Schoen AM. Veterinary acupuncture. Seminars in Veterinary Medicine and Surgery (Small Animal) 1986; 1:224–29.

29. Janssens LA. Trigger points in 48 dogs with myofascial pain syndromes. Vet Surg 1991; 20:274–78.

30. Wright M, McGrath CJ. Physiologic and analgesic effects of acupuncture in the dog. J Am Vet Med Assoc 1981; 178:502–7.

31. American Veterinary Medical Association. Guidelines for alternative and complementary veterinary medicine. AVMA Directory and Resource Manual 46th ed. Schaumburg: Division of Membership and Field Services American Veterinary Medical Association, 1997:55–56.

# Chapter 4 Analgesics and Associated Drugs and Supplements

The analgesics that veterinarians are currently employing in small animal medicine are examined in this chapter. In small animal medicine, analgesics used in the immediate perioperative period generally have been restricted to opioids. Opioids are scheduled drugs; the schedule is essentially determined by the potential for human abuse. The increasing role of local anesthetics and nonsteroidal anti-inflammatory drugs (NSAIDs) in small animal pain management are discussed, as well as the restricted role of the $\alpha_2$-agonists.

There are many published recommendations for dosages of analgesics, with higher dosages being used in animals in severe pain. Generally, the dosages listed in this chapter have been used and found to be appropriate. When a dosage range is provided, usually, the lower dose is administered IV (or at least begun with the lower dosage) and the higher dosages IM or SC. If an intravenous catheter is in place, IV administration avoids painful IM injections. On occasion, veterinarians may administer half of the dosage IV and half SC or IM in order to provide both immediate and sustained analgesia. In the case of drugs that might be useful, but with which experience is limited, the source of the dosage is referenced. When practitioners are determining dosages, they should assess each patient individually and adjust the dosages accordingly.

## Opioids: Agonists, Agonist-Antagonists, Partial Agonists, and Antagonists

*Opioid agonists* stereospecifically bind to opioid receptors to mediate a response. *Opioid antagonists* have a high affinity for opioid receptors and can displace opioid agonists; opioid antagonists have no intrinsic activity so they do not activate opioid receptors, which allows antagonism to occur.[1] *Opioid agonist-antagonists* lack the efficacy of pure agonists, and the antagonist properties of these drugs may attenuate those of subsequently administered pure agonists.[1] The greatest advantage of agonist-antagonists is their ability to produce analgesia with limited respiratory depression. The ceiling effect (administering increasing doses does not produce additional responses) on ventilatory depression is attended by a similar ceiling effect for analgesia (and the ability to decrease anesthetic requirement).[1] Opioid receptors (mu [μ], kappa [κ], delta [δ], sigma [σ]) mediate different responses when activated by an opioid agonist. Since different species respond to opioids in various ways, it is likely that each species has a unique ratio of different receptors, or that receptors mediate different responses in different species. In general, $\mu_1$ receptors are believed to be responsible for supraspinal analgesia and $\mu_2$ receptors for respiratory depression and bradycardia.[1] Delta receptors are believed to modulate μ receptors; k receptors are believed to be responsible for analgesia and some sedation with little effect on ventilation.[1] Sigma receptors are responsible for dysphoria.[1] Different authors[1-3] do not agree on the classification of receptors for all opioid agonists. Pure agonists are generally classified as μ-agonists; agonist-antagonists are generally κ-agonists and μ-antagonists.

### Agonists

The gold standard for comparing analgesics is morphine. When comparing drugs to morphine, veterinarians should consider their efficacy (the magnitude of the maximum effect), onset of action, duration of action, and side effects. Generally, the potency of opioids is also compared to that of morphine. Potency can be misleading since drugs may be many times more potent than morphine, but much less efficacious. The easiest way to think about potency is in terms of the quantity of drug required for an equivalent effect (not how good the drug is for analgesia).

**Morphine**

Morphine, a μ-agonist[1] (also reported as a κ-agonist),[2,3] increases the pain threshold and modifies pain perception. In the absence of pain, it may produce either sedation or dysphoria. Morphine may interact with other drugs to alter hemodynamic parameters.

In people, an overdose of morphine causes death by ventilatory depression.[1] Amphetamines, phenothiazines, monamine oxidase inhibitors, and tricyclic antidepressants enhance the depressant effects of morphine. In dogs and cats, the risk from ventilatory depression, although real, does not appear to be as great as that in people. If ventilatory depression is a concern, oxygen may be insufflated in order to maintain $P_aO_2$ above 80 mm of Hg. Morphine should be used with caution in patients with increased intracranial pressure in which ventilation will not be controlled; hypoventilation (increased $P_aCO_2$ above normal) will increase intracranial pressure.

*Potency*

Morphine is the standard for comparison.

*Efficacy*

Morphine is effective against moderate to severe pain; its greatest efficacy occurs when morphine is given preemptively.

*Side Effects*

Side effects include ventilatory depression, bradycardia, nausea, vomiting, sedation, dysphoria, histamine release (and associated hypotension, urticaria, erythema, pruritus), increased intracranial pressure in the presence of hypoventilation, urinary retention, miosis in dogs, mydriasis in cats, altered temperature regulation (generally causes hypothermia in dogs; may cause hyperthermia in cats), constipation, epigastric pain (biliary smooth muscle spasm), and pancreatic duct smooth muscle contraction.

*Indications*

Morphine is indicated for both visceral and somatic pain. Epidural morphine is appropriate for abdominal procedures and hindlimb procedures. Since morphine is not very lipid soluble and migrates craniad, patients undergoing foreleg amputations and thoracotomies also benefit from receiving epidural morphine.

*Routes of Administration*

Morphine (see Tables 4-1, 4-2, 4-3) may be administered IM, IV, SC, PO, intra-articularly, spinally, and epidurally (use only a preservative-free morphine, such as Duramorph, when administering morphine spinally or epidurally).

In dogs that do not respond to intermittent injections, veterinarians may use morphine as an infusion after a loading dose. The loading dose of morphine in dogs is determined by giving small boluses of morphine (0.1 mg/kg, slowly IV) every 3 to 5 minutes until the desired clinical effect is achieved; be wary of histamine release. Once the loading dose has been determined, the dose may be administered by syringe pump over about 4 hours, or may be added to the fluids to be given over the next 4 hours.[4]

In recent studies, morphine has proven effective when applied to peripheral receptors in canine stifle joints,[5,6] but not when administered interpleurally.[7] Intra-articular morphine (0.1 mg/kg diluted in 1 ml saline/10 kg body weight) was compared to epidural morphine (0.1 mg/kg diluted in 1 ml saline/5 kg body weight).[5] Intra-articular morphine provided analgesia equivalent to epidural morphine.[5] Both groups had lower pain scores than saline-treated groups.[5] Intra-articular morphine (0.1 mg/kg diluted to 0.5 ml saline/kg body weight) or intra-articular bupivacaine (0.5% at 0.5 ml/kg) provided better analgesia than saline in canine stifle surgery, but bupivacaine showed the greatest effect.[6]

Oral forms of morphine, including sustained-release products, are available. Published reports regarding the use of oral morphine in veterinary species are limited.[8–10] Bioavailability of oral sustained-release morphine (1.4 to 2.7 mg/kg) is about 20% in dogs.[9] It appears that twice-daily dosing of oral-sustained release morphine may produce therapeutic morphine concentrations.[9] However, plasma morphine concentrations are poorly correlated with analgesic activity in people, so researchers must still evaluate the therapeutic potential of oral morphine.[9] Begin with the low end of the dose and adjust it for each individual. Empirical doses for standard oral morphine (not sustained-release) of 0.3 to 3 mg/kg, PO every 4 to 8 hours, have been recommended for chronic pain.[10]

*Schedule and Cost*

Morphine is a Schedule II controlled substance. It is the least expensive opioid available.

**Oxymorphone**

Oxymorphone and morphine have similar receptor profiles, onsets, durations, efficacies, uses, and side effects, except for histamine release. The absence of histamine release after IV administration makes oxymorphone attractive for intraoperative management of surgical cases that benefit from low concentrations of inhalant anesthetics supplemented with IV opioids.

*Potency*

Oxymorphone is 10 times as potent as morphine.[1]

*Efficacy*

Same as that for morphine.

*Side Effects*

Same as those for morphine. Intravenous use of oxymorphone is not associated with histamine release. Oxymorphone may cause less vomiting than morphine. Panting is a common sequella, due to resetting of the thermoregulatory center.

*Indications*

Same as those for morphine.

*Routes of Administration*

Oxymorphone may be administered IM, IV, SC (see Tables 4-1 and 4-2), and epidurally (see Table 4-3).

*Schedule and Cost*

Oxymorphone is a Schedule II controlled substance. It is relatively expensive.

**Fentanyl**

Fentanyl and morphine have similar receptor profiles. Fentanyl alone is not approved for use in dogs and cats. Fentanyl is more lipid soluble than morphine; thus, it has a more rapid onset and shorter duration than morphine.[1] Fentanyl is useful for intraoperative management of surgical cases that benefit from minimal concentrations of inhalant anesthetics, supplemented with an opioid. Histamine release after IV fentanyl is insignificant. Although fentanyl is appropriate for moderate to severe pain, the usefulness of fentanyl for analgesia is basically restricted to intravenous constant rate infusion (CRI) due to its very short duration of action. Currently, transcutaneous fentanyl shows

***Table 4-1.** Opioid analgesics for dogs.*

| Drug | Onset IM* (min) | Duration IM* (hr) | Dose and Route† | Indications | Comments |
|---|---|---|---|---|---|
| Morphine | 15 to 30 | 4 | 0.05 to 0.4 mg/kg, IV;‡[4]<br>0.2 to 1.0 mg/kg, SC, IM.[4]<br>See text for oral dosing and CRI. | Moderate to severe pain | Sedation, respiratory depression, bradycardia, nausea, hypothermia |
| Oxymorphone | 20 | 4 | 0.05 to 0.1 mg/kg, IV, SC, IM | Moderate to severe pain | Sedation, respiratory depression, bradycardia, nausea, panting, hypothermia |
| Fentanyl | 10 | <1 | 0.002 to 0.005 mg/kg, IV, IM.§<br>See text for CRI. | Breakthrough pain with concurrent use of fentanyl patch; intraoperative administration; premedicant | Sedation, respiratory depression, bradycardia, nausea; inadequate duration of analgesia from single IV bolus or IM injection |
| Codeine | — | 6 to 8 (oral) | 1 to 2 mg/kg PO<br>(dosed with Tylenol 4).[15]<br>See text for supplemental dosage. | Mild to moderate pain | Minimal side effects.‡ When dosed with Tylenol, avoid in dogs with liver disease or Heinz body anemia |
| Buprenorphine | 30 | 6 to 8 | 0.005 to 0.015 mg/kg, IV, IM | Mild to moderate pain | Prolonged sleep times, vomiting, respiratory depression; difficult to antagonize |
| Butorphanol | 10 to 15 | 1 to 3 | 0.2 to 0.4 mg/kg, IV, SC, IM, PO | Mild to moderate pain‖ | Mild or no sedation, mild ventilatory depression |
| Pentazocine | 15 | 2 | 2 to 3 mg/kg, IM[19] | Mild pain; inadequate for postoperative pain | Mild or no sedation, mild ventilatory depression; dysphoria |

* Onset will be faster and duration shorter when administered IV; generally, onset will be slower and duration longer when administered SC or PO.

† For epidural or spinal use of opioids, see Table 4-3.

‡ Intravenous administration is associated with histamine release.

§ See text for transdermal fentanyl doses.

‖ Clinically, butorphanol appears to be a good analgesic for moderate to severe cranial abdominal pain associated with bile peritonitis or pancreatitis.

**Table 4-2.** *Opioid* analgesics for cats.*

| Drug | Onset IM† (min) | Duration IM† (hr) | Dose and Route‡ | Indications | Comments |
|---|---|---|---|---|---|
| Morphine | 15 to 30 | 4 | 0.05 to 0.2 mg/kg, IM, SC[4] | Moderate to severe pain | Sedation, respiratory depression, bradycardia, nausea, hyperthermia; dysphoria in nonpainful cats or excessive dosage |
| Oxymorphone | 20 | 4 | 0.05 mg/kg, IV, SC, IM | Moderate to severe pain | Sedation, respiratory depression, bradycardia, nausea, hyperthermia; dysphoria in nonpainful cats |
| Buprenorphine | 30 | 6 to 8 | 0.005 to 0.015 mg/kg, IV, IM | Mild to moderate pain | Vomiting, respiratory depression; difficult to antagonize |
| Butorphanol | 10 to 15 | 4 | 0.2 to 0.4 mg/kg, IV, SC, IM, PO | Mild to moderate pain§ | Mild or no sedation, mild ventilatory depression |
| Pentazocine | 15 | 4 to 5 | 2 to 3 mg/kg, IM[19] | Mild pain; inadequate for postoperative pain | Mild or no sedation, mild ventilatory depression; dysphoria |

* See text for transdermal and CRI fentanyl doses.

† Onset will be faster and duration shorter when administered IV. Clinically, IV administration of opioids appears to be more likely to be associated with dysphoria; generally, onset will be slower and duration longer when administered SC or PO.

‡ For epidural or spinal use of opioids, see Table 4-3.

§ Clinically, butorphanol appears to be a good analgesic for moderate to severe pain in some situations for cats.

*Table 4-3.* *Drugs for producing epidural* analgesia or anesthesia in dogs and cats.*

| Drug | Dose† | Onset‡ (min) | Duration‡ (hr) | Indications |
|---|---|---|---|---|
| Morphine§ | Dog and cat: 0.1 mg/kg | 20 | 20 | Analgesia: hindlimb, abdominal, thoracic, and forelimb procedures |
| Oxymorphone | Dog and cat: 0.05 to 0.1 mg/kg[41] | 15‡ | 10 | Analgesia: hindlimb, abdominal procedures |
| Fentanyl | Dog: 0.001 mg/kg | 4 to 10 | 4 to 6[43] | Analgesia: hindlimb, abdominal procedures |
| Buprenorphine | Dog: 0.005 mg/kg | 30‡ | 18 | Analgesia: hindlimb, abdominal procedures |
| Lidocaine 2%‖ | Dog: 1 ml/3.4 kg($T_5$);<br>1 ml/4.5 kg ($L_2$)[41] | 10 | 1 to 1.5 | Anesthesia/analgesia: hindlimb, abdominal procedures |
| | Cat: 1 ml/4.5 kg ($T_5$)[27] | 2 to 10 | 0.75 to 1 | |
| Bupivacaine 0.5%‖ | Dog: 1 ml/4.5 kg<br>Cat: 1 ml/7 kg[27] | 20 to 30<br>15 to 20 | 4.5 to 6<br>3 to 6 | Anesthesia/analgesia: hindlimb, abdominal procedures |

* Decrease the dose by half when administering local anesthetics spinally; decrease the epidural dose in geriatric, obese, and pregnant animals; and in animals with space-occupying lesions of the spinal cord or conditions in which venous engorgement is expected.

† Volume should be below 0.3 ml/kg; do not exceed 6 ml/dog[42] or 1.5 ml/cat (there are other volume recommendations; the author uses these).

‡ When specific onset and duration of action are not known for veterinary patients, they are extrapolated from literature about human patients or from the onset and duration of parenterally administered drugs.

§ Preservative-free morphine (for example, Duramorph) should be used for epidural or spinal administration of morphine.

‖ Avoid head-down positioning of the patient after epidurals; a block to $T_1$ leads to intercostal paralysis, a block to $C_5$–$C_7$ leads to phrenic nerve paralysis.

promise for analgesia in dogs and cats (the technique for fentanyl patch placement is described in chapter 3).

*Potency*

Fentanyl is 75 to 125 times more potent than morphine.[1]

*Efficacy*

Same as that for morphine.

*Side Effects*

Side effects include bradycardia, ventilatory depression, and skeletal muscle rigidity. There is insignificant histamine release.

*Indications*

Same as those for morphine. As an infusion or transdermally, fentanyl may be used for moderate to severe pain. Even though effective as a single injection, it is too short-lived to provide needed perioperative analgesia.

*Routes of Administration*

Fentanyl may be administered IM, SC, IV (see Tables 4-1 and 4-2), transmucosally (lollipop in children), epidurally (see Table 4-3), and transdermally.

For CRI, in dogs, a loading bolus of fentanyl (0.002 mg/kg, IV) is administered and followed by an infusion of 0.001 to 0.006 mg/kg/hr, IV; the duration of analgesia is the duration of the infusion plus 30 minutes.[11] In cats, for CRI, a loading dose of fentanyl (0.001 to 0.002 mg/kg, IV) is followed by an infusion of 0.001 to 0.004 mg/kg/hr; the duration of analgesia is the duration of the infusion plus 30 minutes.[11]

When patches are applied to dogs, approximately 24 hours should be allowed for plasma concentrations to reach steady-state;[12,13] in cats, plasma levels appear to plateau more rapidly.[14] Patches are designed to provide about 72 hours of analgesia, but may be effective for longer periods. Patches are available in 25, 50, 75, and 100 µg/hr concentrations. A patch with 2.5 mg fentanyl is designed to release 25 µg/hr. See chapter 3 for techniques on placing and removing fentanyl patches.

Some caution is necessary when using transdermal fentanyl for analgesia. Therapeutic plasma levels of fentanyl in dogs and cats have not been reliably established. Additionally, there appears to be a great deal of inter- and intraindividual variation in plasma fentanyl concentrations attained after transdermal administration.[12,14] Patients should be evaluated regularly for side effects such as respiratory depression and sedation, as well as for inadequate analgesia; skin irritation from the patch may also occur.[12] The variation of plasma fentanyl concentration may be due to variations in the amount of drug released from the patch, variations in dermal and epidermal uptake (including variations in epidermal thickness), variable cutaneous vasculature uptake, and an individual's metabolic clearance and volume of distribution.[12]

The package insert for transdermal fentanyl patches indicates that patches should not be used for postoperative pain due to serious or life-threatening hypoventilation (Janssen Pharmaceutica, Titusville, NJ, 1994). It should always be remembered that hypoventilation may occur as a result of opioid administration. All postoperative patients should be closely monitored for hypoventilation, but dogs and cats do not seem to be as sensitive to the effects of opioids on ventilation as do people. When a patch is used for chronic pain, the correct patch size will need to be determined by proper dose titration. Additionally, the Drug Enforcement Agency guidelines should be followed when administering scheduled drugs.

The dosage guidelines for fentanyl patches are not well established. Guidelines for fentanyl patch doses based on the body weight of the patient are:

| Patient Weight | Patch Size |
|---|---|
| <3.2 kg (7 pounds) | Not recommended |
| 3.2 to 6.8 kg (7 to 15 pounds) | 25 μg/hr[15] |
| 6.8 to 18.2 kg (15 to 40 pounds) | 50 μg/hr[15] |
| 18.2 to 27.3 kg (40 to 60 pounds) | 75 μg/hr[15] |
| >27.3 kg (60 pounds) | 100 μg/hr[15] |

Since plasma fentanyl concentrations vary greatly in dogs, and larger patches (100 μg/hr) do not appear to increase plasma fentanyl concentrations above those attained with smaller patches (50 μg/hr patches),[12] patients should be closely monitored for signs of analgesic efficacy. In dogs whose patch size is too small to deliver 0.001 to 0.004 mg/kg/hr (1 to 4 μg/kg/hr), alternative analgesic therapy should be available if necessary. Similar problems regarding drug delivery occur with small patients. Veterinarians have tried cutting the patch, or covering a portion of the patch (the amount of patch to be exposed can be calculated by using a dose of 0.004 mg/kg)[14] for smaller patients; however, it is unknown how either method will affect drug delivery.

Breakthrough pain may occur, but in dogs, side effects other than sedation and ataxia are uncommon. In cats, euphoria, purring, and increased appetite may occur; if the absorption rate is too high, dementia, agitation, dilated pupils, and heightened responsiveness may result.[15] As mentioned in chapter 3, fever and contact with warm-water circulating blankets may increase the absorption of fentanyl.

Generally patients are not discharged with fentanyl patches; only patients that the veterinarian has carefully selected should be discharged with patches. In such cases, owners should be advised of the possible behavioral and physiologic side effects and potential adverse consequences for pets or children if they handle or consume a dislodged patch. Veterinarians may want to consider methods to encourage clients to return used patches for proper disposal.

*Schedule and Cost*

Fentanyl is a Schedule II controlled substance. The cost for a transdermal fentanyl patch is reasonable if compared to the cost of 3 days of parenteral opioid therapy.

**Meperidine**

Meperidine and morphine have similar receptor profiles. Meperidine's short duration of action makes it unsatisfactory for analgesia.

*Potency*

Meperidine is $\frac{1}{10}$ as potent as morphine.

*Efficacy*

Same as that for morphine.

*Side Effects*

Side effects include significant hypoventilation, negative inotropy, histamine release, and orthostatic hypotension. Structurally, meperidine is similar to atropine and may produce slight atropine antispasmodic effects, increased heart rate, and dry mouth.[1]

Delirium and seizures may result from accumulation of normeperidine (CNS stimulant).[1]

*Indications*

Meperidine is not indicated for analgesia due to its short duration of action. In dogs and cats, 2 to 5 mg/kg, IM or SC, provides about 1 hour of analgesia.[16]

*Routes of Administration*

Meperidine may be administered IM and IV (consider pretreatment with H-1 and H-2 blockers).

*Schedule and Cost*

Meperidine is a Schedule II controlled substance. It is a relatively inexpensive drug.

**Codeine**

Codeine has a low affinity for opioid receptors and is believed to be analgesic after conversion to morphine.[1] Codeine may be used orally in dogs. Tylenol 4 (60 mg of codeine and 300 mg of acetaminophen) dosed at 1 to 2 mg of codeine/kg of body weight, PO TID, seems safe for healthy dogs[15] (see Table 4-1). Tylenol 4 may be supplemented with codeine alone (1 to 4 mg/kg, PO, between 1 and 6 hours).[4] The codeine-acetominophen combination is strictly contraindicated in cats, and should not be used in dogs with hepatic disease or in dogs prone to Heinz body anemia.[15]

*Potency*

Codeine's potency is as follows: orally, 60 mg codeine = 650 mg aspirin; IM, it is $\frac{1}{12}$ as potent as morphine.[1]

*Efficacy*

Codeine is effective for mild to moderate pain in dogs only.

*Side Effects*

Codeine produces minimal side effects, which are similar to those for morphine; significant histamine release may occur after IV administration of codeine.

*Schedule and Cost*

The schedule of codeine is variable (II to V) depending on the form and concentration. It is relatively inexpensive.

## Agonist-Antagonists and Partial Agonists

The advantage of opioid agonist-antagonists is moderate analgesia, with little ventilatory depression. Agonist-antagonists usually act primarily on k receptors and are less likely to be abused than μ-agonists. The disadvantages are that mixed agonist-antagonists may attenuate the efficacy of subsequently administered agonists and they may cause dysphoria.

**Buprenorphine**

Buprenorphine is variably reported as a partial μ-agonist[2,3] and a κ agonist-antagonist.[1] Its affinity for μ receptors (50 times that of morphine) accounts for its prolonged duration, and difficulty in antagonizing its effects. Antagonist activity is related to its ability to displace more efficacious opioid agonists from μ receptors.[1] The greatest advantage of buprenorphine is its duration of action, which may be 8 hours.

*Potency*

Buprenorphine is about 300 times more potent than morphine.

*Efficacy*

Buprenorphine is effective for mild to moderate pain.

*Side Effects*

Buprenorphine prolongs sleep times, and may induce vomiting and ventilatory depression. Little sedation or dysphoria occurs in dogs and cats as a result of receiving buprenorphine.

*Indications*

Buprenorphine is indicated for prolonged treatment of mild to moderate pain.

*Routes of Administration*

Buprenorphine can be administered IM, IV (see Tables 4-1 and 4-2), and epidurally (see Table 4-3); clinically, SC administration does not appear as efficacious.

*Schedule and Cost*

Buprenorphine is a Schedule V controlled substance. It is relatively inexpensive.

**Butorphanol**

Butorphanol produces analgesia by affecting κ receptors where it has moderate affinity; it produces antagonism at μ receptors where it has a low affinity. There is minimal σ receptor affinity and so very little dysphoria occurs. The ceiling effect (additional doses may not produce additional responses) on ventilation is accompanied by a modest ability to decrease anesthetic requirements (e.g., butorphanol decreases MAC of enflurane only 11% in dogs;[1] butorphanol does not decrease the MAC of halothane in dogs[17]). As a result, intraoperative use of butorphanol as an analgesic during inhalant anesthesia may be limited.

When given the recommended doses of butorphanol, the patient may experience mild to moderate sedation, with a significant degree of variation from patient to patient. When butorphanol is administered preoperatively to nonpainful cats, dysphoria generally does not occur. The greatest disadvantage of butorphanol for perioperative pain management is its short duration of action: In dogs, it lasts 1 to 3 hours; in cats, 4 hours. As a result, redosing is often necessary at extubation. Also, if used with pure opioid agonists, butorphanol may antagonize some of the effects.[1,18]

*Potency*

Butorphanol is 3 to 5 times more potent than morphine and 50 times less potent than naloxone.[19]

*Efficacy*

Butorphanol is effective for mild to moderate pain; visceral analgesia appears to be greater than somatic analgesia.

*Side Effects*

Only occasional vomiting is associated with administration of butorphanol, and respiratory depression appears relatively mild.

*Indications*

Butorphanol is a good analgesic for elective surgical procedures such as neuters, ovariohysterectomies, and onychectomies (see below). In dogs, butorphanol is generally reserved for mild to moderate pain; however, butorphanol appears particularly efficacious for selected cases of moderate to severe cranial abdominal pain, such as bile peritonitis and pancreatitis, perhaps due to its milder effects on the biliary and gastrointestinal tracts.

*Route of Administration*

Butorphanol may be administered IM, IV, SC, or PO (see Tables 4-1 and 4-2).

Butorphanol has been particularly useful for onychectomies in cats; one dose of injectable butorphanol (0.4 mg/kg, IM, SC) is given as a premedicant. Four to 6 hours later, an additional dose is administered SC. The patient is then started on oral butorphanol (usually the next morning) and receives it TID for 2 days. Calculate the oral dose of butorphanol at 0.4 mg/kg; administer either 2.5 mg ($^1/_4$ of a 10-mg tablet) or 5 mg ($^1/_2$ of a 10-mg tablet), whichever is closer to the calculated dose up to 1 mg/kg, TID.

*Schedule and Cost*

Butorphanol is a Schedule IV controlled substance. It is moderately expensive.

**Pentazocine**

Pentazocine is a mixed agonist-antagonist; it is an agonist at $\delta$, $\kappa$, and $\sigma$ receptors. Pentazocine has weak antagonist activity at the μ receptor. It is considered a relatively poor analgesic.

*Potency*

Pentazocine is 0.3 times as potent as morphine.[19]

*Efficacy*

Pentazocine is effective only for mild pain.

*Side Effects*

Side effects include dysphoria and increased plasma concentrations of catecholamines.

*Indications*

Pentazocine is generally not recommended for analgesia, but has been used for mild pain.

*Routes of Administration*

Pentazocine may be administered IM, SC, and PO (see Tables 4-1 and 4-2).

*Schedule and Cost*

Pentazocine is a Schedule IV controlled substance. It is relatively inexpensive.

## Opioid Antagonists

In some circumstances, it will be necessary to antagonize an opioid agonist, especially the μ-agonists. Antagonizing opioids in painful patients (i.e., eliminating analgesia) is not recommended. In people and anecdotally in animals, antagonism of opioids has been associated with endogenous catecholamine release, hypertension, dysrhythmias, and fatalities. If there is a situation in which the cardiopulmonary effects of opioids or opioid combinations are believed to place the patient at risk, antagonism should be undertaken with caution—usually, by slowly titrating the antagonist to produce the specific amount of antagonism desired.

### Nalbuphine

Nalbuphine is a mixed agonist-antagonist, with agonist activity at κ receptors. It is a poor analgesic and its clinical use in veterinary medicine is primarily restricted to reversing the cardiopulmonary depressant effects of μ-agonists while attempting to maintain analgesia. The dose is 0.5 to 1.5 mg/kg, IV, or IM. It is prudent to dilute 1 mg/kg of 20 mg/ml nalbuphine to 10 ml with saline, and titrate it IV to effect. The duration is believed to be 3 to 8 hours,[20] but patients should be monitored for renarcotization.

### Naloxone

Naloxone is a relatively pure μ-antagonist. Naloxone is used to reverse ventilatory depression or excessive sedation. It has a short duration of action (about 20 minutes in dogs), so repeated dosing may be necessary to sustain antagonism. High doses have been used to treat hypovolemic shock, and to a lesser extent septic shock. Reversal of analgesia is perhaps the worst side effect of naloxone in painful patients. Increased sympathetic tone associated with the administration of naloxone may cause cardiovascular stimulation. Tachycardia, hypertension, pulmonary edema, cardiac dysrhythmias, and ventricular fibrillation have been reported.[1] Nausea and vomiting may occur.[1] The dose is 0.02 mg/kg, IM, SC, IV, or half IV and half SC in dogs and cats. It is advisable to draw up 1 ml (0.4 mg) and dilute it with 9 ml of saline, and titrate it IV to effect.

## Dissociative Anesthetics

*Dissociative anesthetics* produce a cataleptic state in which the eyes are open. Generally, animals receiving dissociatives are immobilized, but varying degrees of skeletal muscle movement may occur.[1] Dissociatives produce amnesia and analgesia.[1] Somatic analgesia may be profound; however, visceral analgesia is limited.

### Ketamine

In dogs and cats, ketamine at low dosages (0.5 to 1.0 mg/kg, IM) may be used to provide somatic analgesia without cataleptoid effects or unconsciousness; 1 to 2 mg/kg, IV, or 2 to 4 mg/kg, IM, IV, may provide 30 minutes of analgesia.[16] Ketamine provides little visceral analgesia.[21] Ketamine is excreted unchanged by the kidneys in cats[22] and should not be used in cats with primary renal disease.

*Side Effects*

The side effects of ketamine are dose related and include emergence delirium, cardiovascular stimulation (increased heart rate and blood pressure), increased intracranial pressure, increased intraocular pressure, seizures, increased salivation and lacrimation, and bronchodilation.

*Indications*

Ketamine may be used as an analgesic treatment for burns and wounds.

*Routes of Administration*

Ketamine may be administered IM or IV.

*Schedule and Cost*

Ketamine is currently not scheduled in most states and is relatively inexpensive; it may become a scheduled drug.

## Alpha$_2$-Agonists

Alpha$_2$-agonists (e.g., xylazine, medetomidine) have profound cardiopulmonary effects in dogs and cats. Their sedative effects generally outlast their analgesic effects. Although these drugs are appropriate for sedation and chemical restraint, due to their cardiovascular effects, their use in perioperative analgesia is often limited to young, healthy dogs and cats. If $\alpha_2$-agonists are used as part of the anesthetic regimen, adding opioid analgesics may potentiate cardiopulmonary depression. Butorphanol may be added postoperatively to an anesthetic regimen utilizing $\alpha_2$-agonists for analgesia since it has relatively mild cardiopulmonary side effects. If butorphanol is used preoperatively, the dose of $\alpha_2$-agonist administered may generally be decreased and the combined effect will be sedation and analgesia.

Caution has been advocated when using $\alpha_2$-agonists as postoperative analgesics and anxiolytics since postsurgical doses and duration are not well established and profound cardiac depressant effects may occur.[11] Anticholinergics frequently need to be administered. Xylazine (0.1 to 1 mg/kg, IV, IM, SC) has been used in dogs and cats to provide analgesia for acute pain for 0.5 to 2 hours.[11] As a postoperative sedative, xylazine (0.1 to 0.5 mg/kg, IV, IM, SC) has been used for postoperative anxiety.[11] Medetomidine (0.001 to 0.01 mg/kg, IV, IM, SC) has been used for postoperative analgesia for 0.5 to 2 hours in dogs and cats with acute pain.[11] As a postoperative anxiolytic, medetomidine at lower doses (0.001 to 0.005 mg/kg, IV, IM, SC) has been used.[11] Higher doses of medetomidine have been examined as a preanesthetic and as a sole agent for sedation and analgesia in dogs.[23]

Special care should be taken when antagonizing $\alpha_2$-agonists, particularly in painful patients, since analgesia will also be reversed. Antagonizing $\alpha_2$-agonists with $\alpha_2$-antagonists (e.g., yohimbine, tolazoline, atipamezole) reverses the cardiopulmonary, sedative, and analgesic effects of $\alpha_2$-agonists. Sympathetic stimulation, which occurs with the sudden onset of pain, may have cardiopulmonary consequences (see discussion of antagonism of opioid agonists earlier in this chapter).

## Steroids

Glucocorticoids inhibit the arachadonic acid cascade, and have anti-inflammatory, antipyretic, and analgesic effects. Corticosteroids inhibit phospholipase $A_2$, thereby limiting production of arachadonic acid.[24] Arachadonic acid is the precursor of both prostaglandins, which lower nociceptive thresholds, and leukotrines, which cause hyperalgesia. [24] Corticosteroids may reduce bone pain,[10] increase appetite and weight gain, and produce polyuria and polydipsia. Corticosteroids have been historically used to treat osteoarthritis.[24] Long-term use of parenteral corticosteroids may cause iatrogenic hyperadrenocorticism. Intra-articular administration of corticosteroids may potentially accelerate cartilage damage and may precipitate adverse systemic affects.[24] Corticosteroids should not be used in conjunction with NSAIDs due to the increased risk of gastrointestinal ulceration and perforation.

## Nonsteroidal Anti-Inflammatory Drugs (NSAIDS)

The mechanism of action of NSAIDs[24] and currently available NSAIDs[25] have recently been reviewed; the interested reader is encouraged to consult these articles for details not discussed in this text.[24,25] NSAIDs suppress prostaglandin synthesis by blocking cyclooxygenase (COX), which transforms arachadonic acid to prostaglandins.[25] Prostaglandins lower the nociceptive threshold to agents like bradykinin, serotonin, and histamine.[25] Additionally, NSAIDs inhibit neutrophil activation. They produce analgesia and reduce inflammation. Inflammation and tissue trauma amplify nociception, and NSAIDs prevent that amplification.[26]

In the past, NSAIDs have been used in dogs to control mild to moderate chronic pain, but they have not been relied on for perioperative analgesia until recently. Nonsteroidal anti-inflammatory agents have not been used extensively in cats due to toxicity. However, the newer NSAIDs include drugs that are more efficacious analgesics with fewer side effects. As a result, they are being used more in the perioperative period in dogs. Recently, newer NSAIDs with fewer gastrointestinal and renal side effects are being used in cats. Even so,

NSAIDs should only be used in healthy, young, normotensive, normovolemic dogs and cats with no evidence of gastric ulceration, bleeding diathesis, or compromised renal function.

Gastrointestinal disorders are the most common side effect of NSAIDs.[24] Recent evidence helps to explain why some drugs produce more adverse gastrointestinal effects than others. There are two isoforms of COX: COX-1, the constitutive form (important in maintaining physiologic homeostasis[24] through production of physiologically cytoprotective prostaglandins),[25] and COX-2, the inducible form.[24] COX-1 is found in stomach, kidney, endothelium, and platelets; COX-2 is believed to be produced by cells in association with inflammation.[24] NSAIDs inhibit COX-1 and COX-2; dexamethasone inhibits only COX-2.[24] The current thinking is that agents with higher COX-1 specificity result in greater gastrointestinal injury;[24] drugs with more selectivity for COX-2 than for COX-1 result in less gastrointestinal injury.[24] For example, meloxicam, an NSAID licensed in Europe (currently not available in the United States), repeatedly produces greater activity against COX-2 than COX-1.[25]

It may be prudent for veterinarians to add drugs for prophylaxis and treatment of ulcers to the NSAIDs regimen (see below). If ulcer prophylaxis is used in cats, care should be taken to avoid constipation. Although not a common practice yet, it may be best to reserve NSAIDs for supplementing patients that are still painful after receiving an opioid. NSAIDs should not be used in conjunction with corticosteroids. Using NSAIDs preemptively may also be questionable since both increased hemorrhage and renal damage (if patients become hypotensive) may occur intraoperatively.

In human medicine, there are responders and nonresponders to different NSAIDs.[26] If one agent does not produce the desired clinical effect, the physician may try a different agent. Since the mechanism of action is not completely understood, different drugs in the same class or drugs from different classes may be effective. Dogs and cats are particularly sensitive to NSAIDs; caregivers should not use an individual NSAID unless they have evidence that it is safe and efficacious. NSAIDs are not true prostaglandin antagonists because the prostaglandins that are released before the NSAID is administered will continue to exert an effect for some time. In patients with preexisting trauma, the NSAID's effect may not be apparent until the activity of the inflammatory mediators already released has stopped.[26]

**Aspirin**

Historically, aspirin (a salicylate) has been used in dogs at 10 mg/kg, PO, every 12 hours. In cats, 10 mg/kg, PO, may be administered every 48 hours.[27] Aspirin has been recommended for use in cats with osteoarthritis.[28] Aspirin is associated with gastrointestinal lesions and is chondrodestructive.[25]

**Phenylbutazone**

Phenylbutazone (a pyrazole derivative) has been used in dogs at 10 to 20 mg/kg, PO, every 8 hours or 5 to 10 mg/kg, IV, every 8 hours.[27] A maximum of 800 mg/day has been recommended.[4] Administering phenylbutazone to cats is not advised. Phenylbutazone may be associated with anorexia, emesis, depression, and death in cats.[19] Phenylbutazone is associated with gastrointestinal lesions and bone marrow suppression, and is chondrodestructive.[25]

**Flunixin**

Flunixin (a nicotinic acid derivative) has been used to control surgical pain in dogs at 1.0 mg/kg, IV, SC, or IM, daily and in cats at 0.25 mg/kg, SC or IM.[29] Although flunixin may be repeated once in 12 to 24 hours in cats, a onetime IM dose only is recommended.[29] Some risks exist if flunixin is used perioperatively in dogs and cats. Postoperative flunixin (1 mg/kg, IV) has been advocated as a treatment for postoperative pain in dogs either alone or as an adjunct to opioid analgesia; it compared favorably to postoperative treatment with papaveretum (0.2 mg/kg, IV);[30] papaveretum has the analgesic properties of morphine. Reid and Nolan[30] recommended using flunixin for only 3 days because of the potential for gastrointestinal and renal toxicity; nephrotoxicity may develop with methoxyflurane.[30] Flunixin (1 mg/kg, IV) was used in 18 cats undergoing different orthopedic and soft-tissue surgeries.[31] Postoperative analgesia appeared adequate and without untoward side effects.[31] However, until larger studies that document minimal side effects are undertaken, practitioners should administer flunixin cautiously in the perioperative period, and they should not use it preemptively in dogs and cats.

**Ketoprofen**

Ketoprofen (a propionic acid derivative) is a relatively new NSAID. An initial dose of 2.0 mg/kg, IV, SC, or IM, in dogs[29] and a 2.0 mg/kg dose, SC, in cats[29,32] have been recommended. Subsequently, 1 mg/kg daily, PO,[29] may be administered in dogs and cats. Vomiting may occur.[29] Ketoprofen is associated with gastrointestinal lesions but is probably chondroprotective.[25] In a study of orthopedic hindlimb surgery, dogs that received ketoprofen (2.0 mg/kg, IM) had longer and greater analgesia than dogs that received oxymorphone alone, butorphanol alone, or ketoprofen (2.0 mg/kg, IM) and oxymorphone, except during the first postsurgical hour.[33]

**Carprofen**

Carprofen (a carbazole derivative) has been associated with fewer gastrointestinal side effects than other NSAIDs since carprofen's mode of action is believed to be other than cyclooxygenase or 12-lipoxygenase inhibition. An injectable form is available in some countries, and dosage recommendations have been made.[29] For example, 4 mg/kg, SC (once only), is the approved dose for cats in Europe. In cats, 4 mg/kg, SC, administered at extubation provided better analgesia than pethidine (meperidine: 10 mg/kg, IM) from 2 to 20 hours postoperatively without affecting renal function.[34] However, only the oral form of carprofen is available in the United States at this time. In dogs, 2.2 mg/kg of carprofen, PO BID, may be administered. Postoperative analgesia from carprofen has been compared to that found with pethidine[35] and papaveretum[36] in dogs. In dogs undergoing orthopedic procedures, preoperative carprofen (4.0 mg/kg, SC) provided slightly better analgesia and less sedation than preoperative pethidine (2 mg/kg, IM) combined with postoperative pethidine (3 mg/kg, IM).[35] In dogs undergoing orthopedic and soft-tissue surgeries, carprofen (4 mg/kg, IV) produced analgesia as effectively as papaveretum (0.2 mg/kg, IV) administered within 35 minutes of anesthetic induction, but analgesia lasted longer with carprofen.[36]

Carprofen has a high safety profile in dogs.[25] Based on information that the pharmaceutical company provided, there have been isolated reports of hepatic disease occurring in Labrador Retrievers and perhaps other breeds receiving carprofen chronically (letter from Pfizer to veterinarians, 7/30/97). The patients recovered after they received supportive therapy and stopped receiving the drug; the problem is being investigated (letter from Pfizer to veterinarians, 7/30/97).

**Ketorolac**

Ketorolac (an acetic acid derivative) is available in injectable and oral formulations. In dogs, 0.3 to 0.5 mg/kg, IV or IM, may be given every 8 to 12 hours for one to two treatments; in cats, 0.25 mg/kg, IM, every 8 to 12 hours for one to two treatments may be administered.[29] There is a strong potential for gastric ulcers; if ketorolac is selected, the potential benefit should outweigh the risks; ketorolac is probably safer than flunixin.[29]

**Meclofenamic Acid**

Meclofenamic acid (a fenamate derivative) is approved for use in dogs; 1.1 mg/kg, PO, may be administered every 24 hours. Meclofenamic acid is a potent cyclooxygenase inhibitor, and its use may be associated with gastrointestinal disorders.

**Dimethyl Sulfoxide (DMSO)**

DMSO has been used topically and parenterally as an analgesic anti-inflammatory, but is approved only for topical use. DMSO can facilitate transport of low molecular substances through mucous membranes and intact skin. There are many reported actions of DMSO and its metabolite, including reduction of nociceptive impulse conduction. There are few controlled studies demonstrating its usefulness, but DMSO has a wide range of side effects, including hemolysis, diuresis, tertatogenicity, and immunosuppression.[37]

**Prophylaxis and Treatment of Gastrointestinal Ulceration**

Several options have been suggested for the prophylaxis and treatment of ulcers associated with NSAIDs. Some of these regimens include constipating drugs. Such drugs should be used cautiously in cats, and only if the potential benefit outweighs the potential for harm. Sucralfate binds to mucosal defects, providing a barrier to gastric acid; it may prevent signs of GI ulceration and accelerates healing.[29] Ranitidine may be protective against duodenal ulcers.[29] Misoprostol enhances natural mucosal defense mechanisms and helps to prevent ulcers.[29] If the two drugs are administered in the same patient, misoprostol should be given 1 hour before or 2 hours after sucralfate.[29] Misoprostol should be used with caution in patients with a history of epileptic seizures.[29]

*Dosages for Anti-Ulcer Preparations for Dogs and Cats*

| Drug | Dogs | Cats |
|---|---|---|
| Sucralfate | 0.5 to 1.0 g, PO TID[29] | 0.25 g, PO BID or TID[29] |
| Ranitidine | 1 to 2 mg/kg, PO, or 0.5 to 1.0 mg/kg, IV BID[29] | 3.5 mg/kg, PO BID, or 2.5 mg/kg, IV BID[29] |
| Misoprostol | 2 to 5 μg/kg, PO TID[29] | 1 to 3 μg/kg, PO (Boothe, personal communication) |

## Local Anesthetics

Veterinarians frequently select local anesthetics to provide analgesia for surgical procedures in dogs and cats. Neural blockade may be used to decrease postoperative morbidity by enhancing postoperative analgesia. Neural blockade will prevent acute pain; intermittently administering local anesthetics will interrupt sensory transmission. However, regional nerve blocks are not specific for pain fibers and usually affect noxious, sympathetic, and motor activity. Specific contraindications for local anesthetics, reasons for varying the dose, and how to perform techniques are covered in chapter 3 and Appendix A.

Dosing of local anesthetics for neural blockade in dogs and particularly in cats should be based on an accurate weight. Hall and Clark[38] suggest that 10 mg/kg of lidocaine may be infiltrated before toxic signs are visible. Rarely would it be necessary to exceed 6 mg/kg of lidocaine for infiltration in dogs. Veterinarians have long believed that cats may be more sensitive to the toxic side effects of local anesthetics than are dogs. Chadwick[39] demonstrated the mean convulsive dose of lidocaine to be 11.7 mg/kg ± 4.6 mg/kg, IV, and of bupivacaine to be 3.8 mg/kg ± 1.0 mg/kg, IV, in cats; the mean cardiotoxic dose was higher. ECG changes were apparent before EEG changes in both groups, although rarely in the lidocaine group.[39]

Bupivacaine is usually the drug of choice for providing long-lasting local anesthesia. Even though the onset of action with bupivacaine is slower than with lidocaine, bupivacaine's duration is much longer (4 to 8 hours). In dogs, the total dose of bupivacaine should not exceed 2 mg/kg; it is often diluted with saline, depending on where it is used. Generally, the total dose of bupivacaine should not exceed 0.5 to 1 mg/kg in cats.

Lidocaine or bupivacaine may be used for epidural anesthesia in dogs and cats (see Table 4-3). For other local anesthetic techniques, determine the maximum dose of local anesthetic, and do not exceed that dose; sufficient contact time (20 minutes for bupivacaine) must be allowed.

## Examples of Local Anesthetic Doses

For onychectomies in cats, the maximum dose of bupivacaine is calculated and divided among 10 toes. For a 1.4-kg (3-pound) kitten, 0.25 ml of 0.5% (1.25 mg) bupivacaine will allow one drop per toe from a tuberculin syringe without a needle. [An alternative for onychectomies is a ring block at the level of the carpus (P. Hellyer, personal communication).]

For intercostal anesthesia, between 0.25 ml of 0.5% bupivacaine/site (for cats)[27] and 0.5 ml of 0.5% bupivacaine/site (for larger dogs) may be administered. For interpleural anesthesia, do not exceed 2 mg/kg of bupivacaine in dogs; the drug may be diluted with saline to increase volume. For interpleural anesthesia in cats, 0.075 ml of 0.5% bupivacaine/kg body weight (0.375 mg/kg) should be diluted in 2.5 to 5 ml saline for administration in the thorax.[27] If intercostal and interpleural blocks are both employed to provide analgesia for a thoracotomy, the dose should be adjusted to maintain total dose below 2 mg/kg in dogs and below 0.5 to 1 mg/kg in cats.

For canine stifle surgery, intra-articular bupivacaine (0.5 ml of 0.5%/kg) provides analgesia.[6]

In unremitting pain, lidocaine infusions, at 20 μg/kg/minute, IV, may be used in conjunction with other nonlocal anesthetic analgesic techniques for dogs.

## Nutraceuticals

Nutraceuticals with glycosaminoglycans and chondroitin are becoming more popular for use in chronic inflammatory conditions such as arthritis in dogs and cats. There are limited controlled studies in veterinary patients. Currently, some individuals respond well; others appear to have little response. Usually, it takes from weeks to months to see improvement, so their use in acute pain management is limited. For dogs and cats with chronic arthritis, it may be worthwhile to try one of the products; if the patient responds positively, there are generally few attendant untoward effects. As stated in chapter 3, the guidelines for alternative and complementary veterinary care[40] should govern how veterinarians use nutraceuticals. The guidelines indicate that veterinarians should use micronutrients, macronutrients, and nutritional supplements under a valid veterinarian/client/patient relationship, and that they should communicate the risks and benefits; continuing research and education are advised.[40]

## Miscellaneous Drugs

Several drugs are not analgesics but may be used to manage acutely painful patients. Tranquilizers such as acepromazine or diazepam should not be used alone in painful animals. After receiving adequate analgesia, some dogs and cats will continue to show some excitement; in such cases, it is then appropriate to tranquilize the patient.

### Acepromazine

Acepromazine is an excellent anxiolytic; however, it is not a benign drug. Acepromazine should not be used in patients with hypovolemia, a history of seizures, or clotting disorders. It has a long duration of action, and there is no antagonist. In nonpainful dogs and cats, use 0.05 mg/kg, SC, IM, or IV, and do not exceed a total dose of 1 mg.

### Diazepam

Diazepam has few cardiopulmonary effects, but is not a very good anxiolytic in veterinary medicine. It is unreliable for sedation, and may excite patients. Diazepam is a more reliable sedative in old or sick dogs and cats. In nonpainful dogs and cats, use 0.2 mg/kg, IV. Diazepam can be antagonized with flumazenil (0.011 to 0.022 mg/kg, IV,[41] titrated to effect).

## References


1. Stoelting RK. Opioid agonists and antagonists. In: Pharmacology and physiology in anesthetic practice. Philadelphia: J. B. Lippincott Company 1987:69–101.
2. Raffe MR, Tranquilli WJ. Classifying commonly used analgesic agents. Vet Med 1989; 84:687–90.
3. Bednarski RM. Anesthesia and pain control. Vet Clin No Am: Sm An Prac 1989; 19:1223–38.
4. Hansen B. Analgesic therapy. Compendium Continuing Educ Practicing Vet 1994; 16:868–75.
5. Day TK, Pepper WT, Tobias TA, Flynn MF, Clarke KM. Comparison of intra-articular and epidural morphine for analgesia following stifle arthotomy in dogs. Vet Surg 1995; 24:522–30.
6. Sammarco JL, Conzemius MG, Perkowski SZ, Weinstein MJ, Gregor TP, Smith GK. Postoperative analgesia for stifle surgery: a comparison of intra-articular bupivacaine, morphine, or saline. Vet Surg 1996; 25:59–69.
7. Stobie D, Caywood DD, Rozanski EA, et al. Evaluation of pulmonary function and analgesia in dogs after intercostal thoracotomy and use of morphine administered intramuscularly or intrapleurally and bupivacaine administered intrapleurally. Am J Vet Res 1995; 56:1098–1109.
8. Flecknell PA. The relief of pain in laboratory animals. Laboratory Animals 1984; 18:147–60.
9. Dohoo S, Tasker RAR, Donald A. Pharmacokinetics of parenteral and oral sustained-release morphine. J Vet Pharmacol Therap 1994; 17:426–33.
10. Kyles AE. Clinical pain management. Perspectives March/April 1995:6–12.
11. Hellyer PW, Gaynor JS. Acute postsurgical pain in dogs and cats. Compendium Continuing Educ Practicing Vet 1998; 20:140–53.
12. Egger CM, Duke T, Archer J, Cribb PH. Comparison of plasma fentanyl concentrations by using three transdermal fentanyl patch sizes in dogs. Vet Surg 1998; 27:159–66.
13. Kyles AE, Papich M, Hardie EM. Disposition of transdermally administered fentanyl in dogs. Am J Vet Res 1996; 57:715–9.
14. Scherk-Nixon M. A study of the use of a transdermal fentanyl patch in cats. J Am Anim Hosp Assoc 1996; 32:19–24.
15. Hansen B. How to prevent and relieve patient pain. Vet Forum 1996; 13:34–9.
16. Tranquilli WJ, Fikes LL, Raffe MR. Selecting the right analgesics: indications and dosage requirements. Vet Med 1989; 84:692–97.
17. Quandt JE, Raffe R, Robinson EP. Butorphanol does not reduce the minimal alveolar concentration of halothane in dogs. Vet Surg 1994; 23:156–59.
18. McCrackin MA, Harvey RC, Sackman JE, McLean RA, Paddleford RR. Butorphanol tartrate for partial reversal of oxymorphone-induced postoperative respiratory depression in the dog. Vet Surg 1994; 23:67–74.
19. Sackman JE. Pain. Part II. Control of pain in animals. Compendium Continuing Educ Practicing Vet 1991; 13:181–93.
20. Jenkins WJ. Pharmacologic aspects of analgesic drugs in animals: an overview. J Am Vet Med Assoc 1987; 191:1231–40.

21. Sawyer DC, Rech RH, Durham RA. Does ketamine provide adequate visceral analgesia when used alone or in combination with acepromazine, diazepam, or butorphanol in cats? J Am Anim Hosp Assoc 1993; 29:257–63.
22. Haskins SC, Peiffer RL, Stowe CM. A clinical comparison of CT1341, ketamine, and xylazine in cats. Am J Vet Res 1975; 36:1537–43.
23. Short CE. Comparative biochemical and neurologic responses: $\alpha_2$-adrenergic agonist analgesia and anesthesia. In: The effects of selective $\alpha_2$-adrenoceptor agonists on cardiovascular and pulmonary functions and brain wave activity in dogs and horses. Santa Barbara: Veterinary Practice Publishing Company, 1991.
24. Johnston SA, Fox SM. Mechanisms of action of anti-inflammatory medications used for the treatment of osteoarthritis. J Am Vet Med Assoc 1997; 210:1486–92.
25. Fox SM, Johnston SA. Use of carprofen for the treatment of pain and inflammation in dogs. J Am Vet Med Assoc 1997; 210: 1493–98.
26. Lee VC, Rowlingson JC. Pre-emptive analgesia: update on nonsteroidal anti-inflammatory drugs in anesthesia. St. Louis: Mosby, 1995:69–110.
27. Robinson EP. Preoperative and postoperative pain control in the dog and cat. In: Animal pain and its control. Proceedings 226 in conjunction with the Chapter of Anaesthetics and Intensive Care of the Australian College of Veterinary Scientists. Sydney: Post Graduate Committee in Veterinary Science University of Sydney, 1994:423–39.
28. Boothe DM. Medical management of osteoarthritis. In: Proceedings. 14th Annual ACVIM Forum 1996; 274–77.
29. Mathews KA. Nonsteroidal antiinflammatory analgesics to manage acute pain in dogs and cats. Compendium Continuing Educ Practicing Vet 1996; 18:1117–23.
30. Reid J, Nolan AM. A comparison of the postoperative analgesic and sedative effects of flunixin and papaveretum in the dog. J Sm Anim Prac 1991; 32:603–8.
31. Fonda D. Postoperative analgesic effect of flunixin in the cat. J Vet Anaesth 1993; 20:29.
32. Brearley JC. Sedation, premedication and analgesia. In: Hall LW, Taylor P, eds. Anaesthesia of the Cat. London: Bailliere Tindall, 1994:111–28.
33. Pibarot R, Dupuis J, Grisneaux E, et al. Comparison of ketoprofen, oxymorphone hydrochloride, and butorphanol in the treatment of postoperative pain in dogs. J Am Vet Med Assoc 1997; 211:438–44.
34. Lascelles BDX, Cripps P, Mirchandani S, Waterman AE. Carprofen as an analgesic for postoperative pain in cats: dose titration and assessment of efficacy in comparison to pethidine hydrochloride. J Sm Anim Pract 1995; 36:535–41.
35. Lascelles BDX, Butterworth SJ, Waterman AE. Postoperative analgesic and sedative effects of carprofen and pethidine in dogs. Vet Rec 1994; 134:187–91.
36. Nolan A, Reid J. Comparison of the postoperative analgesic and sedative effects of carprofen and papaveretum in the dog. Vet Rec 1993; 133:240–42.

37. Dart CM. The basis for the use of steroids/nonsteroidal anti-inflammatory drugs (NSAID) for pain in clinical practice. In: Animal pain and its control. Proceedings 226 in conjunction with the Chapter of Anaesthetics and Intensive Care of the Australian College of Veterinary Scientists. Sydney: Post Graduate Committee in Veterinary Science University of Sydney, 1994:351–66.

38. Hall LW, Clarke KW. General principles of local analgesia. In: Veterinary anaesthesia. 9th ed. London: Bailliere Tindall, 1991:173–88.

39. Chadwick HS. Toxicity and resuscitation in lidocaine- or bupivacaine-infused cats. Anesthesiology 1985; 63:385–90.

40. American Veterinary Medical Association. Guidelines for alternative and complementary veterinary medicine. AVMA Directory and Resource Manual 46th ed. Schaumburg, Division of Membership and Field Services American Veterinary Medical Association 1997:55–56.

41. Muir WW, Hubbell JAE. Handbook of Veterinary Anesthesia. St. Louis: CV Mosby Co, 1995, 2nd ed.

42. Pascoe PJ. Advantages and guidelines for using epidural drugs for analgesia. Vet Clin No Am: Sm An Prac 1992; 22:421–24.

43. McMurphy RM. Postoperative epidural analgesia. Vet Clin No Am: Sm An Prac 1993; 23:703–16.

# Chapter 5 Monitoring Analgesic Therapy

How can success in treating patients in pain be monitored? Veterinarians can use the same parameters they used to determine if the patient needed analgesic therapy. Generally, surgical patients should be treated for pain for 1 to 3 days postoperatively; treatment duration for patients with painful medical conditions should be determined by the progress of their disease. It may be difficult to accurately assess the presence of pain in a heavily sedated or tranquilized animal. As the effects of sedatives, tranquilizers, and anesthetics decrease with time (or if analgesics that do not cause sedation are used) it usually becomes easier to accurately assess patient status.

## Physiologic Signs

Pain may be present if a patient has an increased heart rate, increased blood pressure, cardiac arrhythmias, labored or shallow breathing, pale mucous membranes, dilated pupils, increased body temperature, salivation, or a combination of these physiologic signs. In general, body systems should normalize after pain is treated, assuming that the patient is physiologically normal in most respects. Heart rate should be within normal limits, pulse quality should be strong, and blood pressure should be within the normal range for the particular species. Respiratory rate and pattern should be normal; shallow breathing should not occur; panting may occur in some dogs treated with opioids, particularly oxymorphone. Blood pressure should be within normal limits; measuring the indirect systolic blood pressure has been a particularly useful technique in identifying painful cats.[1] The mucous membranes should be pink and the capillary refill time should be less than 2 seconds. Pale mucous membranes may indicate vasoconstriction associated with endogenous release of catecholamines, brick-red mucous membranes may indicate $CO_2$ retention associated with ineffective ventilation, and cyanotic mucous membranes may be associated with hypoxemia. In instances of cranial abdominal pain or thoracic pain, ineffective coughing may cause secretion retention. Atelectasis, secretion retention, and subsequent infection may result in hypercarbia and hypoxemia; effective analgesia may protect against these problems. Since thermoregulation may be compromised in patients treated with tranquilizers or analgesics, body temperature should be monitored and supported if necessary. Caution is advised when using external heat sources or cooling devices for patients that are sedated; the sedated patient may be unable or unwilling to move from an environment that is uncomfortable, and the caregiver must ensure the patient's safety. External heat sources, especially heating lamps, may cause full-thickness skin burns.

Generally, qualitative assessment of these physiologic variables when used in conjunction with other indicators of pain will be sufficient to guide therapeutic decisions. However, in some cases, it is helpful to quantify changes in physiologic variables. For example, increases in physiologic variables above a presurgical value may be quantified and assigned a score (e.g., 0 to 15% above presurgical values receives a score of 0; >45% above presurgical values receives a score of 3).[2] The goal of therapy is to minimize the score. These scores can be used in conjunction with subjective behavioral scores (discussed below) to adjust therapy.

Additional physiologic variables should be monitored as indicated by the patient's status. For example, arterial blood gases should be used to evaluate ventilation and oxygenation in patients with suspected ventilatory compromise. Pulse oximetry may be used in respiratory patients that will tolerate placement of a probe on the tongue; if necessary, alternative sites (e.g., the ear, toe web, tail) may be used to monitor trends (see Figure 6-3). Glucose concentration should be evaluated in patients that may be hypoglycemic (e.g., sepsis); elevated glucose concentrations may indicate ongoing stress. Packed cell volume and total solids should be measured to evaluate blood loss and hydration status. The patient should be weighed daily for assessment of hydration status and weight loss. Intravenous fluids should be administered as necessary to support circulating fluid volume. If urinary retention is suspected, the bladder should be palpated; if urine is being retained, the bladder should be expressed regularly, or a urinary catheter should be considered. The size of the bladder should be checked in any animal that received an epidural. Overdistension of the bladder is a possible cause of abnormal heart rates and should be considered when assessing the presence of pain.

Additional parameters should be evaluated if NSAIDs are being administered. The patient should be observed for vomiting and diarrhea. The stool may be checked for blood (melena). It may also be appropriate to monitor renal and hepatic function in patients receiving NSAIDs. Mucosal bleeding time and a clotting profile may be evaluated if impaired platelet function or hemostasis is suspected.

The patient should be arousable even during treatment with analgesics that cause sedation. As lingering anesthetic effects dissipate, the comfortable patient should be aware of its environment. The patient should be interested in the happenings in its surroundings and in interactions with its caretakers. For example, the patient should greet caregivers normally when they approach the cage. The patient should ingest normal amounts of food and water; nutrition is important during healing and caregivers should encourage the patient to consume an adequate amount of calories. Cats should use their litter boxes; dogs should not have breaks in house-training. The animals should groom themselves. Activity level should return to normal, with the usual restrictions on movement (e.g., walking with a leash, or in the case of cats, restricted jumping and climbing); pain should not be used to restrict activity.

To limit activity, environmental confinement should be attempted first (cage enclosure or a kennel). Tranquilizers or sedatives may be necessary for particularly active dogs. The cat illustrated in Figure 2-1 A shows no interest in its surroundings, in eating or drinking, or in activity. In Figures 2-1 B and 2-1 C, one can see marked improvement; the cat is alert and comfortable 16 hours after surgery and a morphine epidural.

## Pain Scoring Techniques

All behavioral pain scoring techniques (simple descriptive scale, numerical rating score, visual analog score) are subject to criticism.[3] A reliable, sensitive, specific scale without variability among observers has not been determined for veterinary patients.[3] Given that there are limitations to different subjective measurements of pain[3] and that subjective behavioral signs are unique for each animal,[4] it may be helpful for veterinarians to assign a pain score when beginning to evaluate a patient's behavior. The scoring systems (see Tables 5-1 and 5-2) shown here have been used in clinical research to examine analgesic efficacy. They are not meant to replace clinical judgment or to deny treatment. These scores are intended to be a beginning to direct attention to changes in posture, response to palpation, appetite, and attitude. Each table can be individualized for different surgeries. Well-controlled pain threshold tests (e.g., decrease in the amount of force applied to a painful area before eliciting a response) tend to be excellent measures of the severity of pain,[4] and can be incorporated into the scale.

Owners may use similar scoring systems. Owners may contribute a great deal of information regarding the postoperative comfort of patients at home. Owners have successfully used an appetite scoring system, a personality scoring system, and a lameness scoring system (see Figure 5-1) to evaluate postoperative comfort in their cats after an onychectomy.

Stress-related hormones and metabolites—including epinephrine, norepinephrine, β-endorphins, free fatty acids, and cortisol—are not practical for evaluating analgesia and pain in individual clinical cases. Individuals vary enormously in resting concentrations of these

***Table 5-1.*** *Scoring system used to evaluate analgesia in dogs after an ear ablation. Adapted from Buback et al.*[5] *and Hardie et al.*[6]

| Analgesia score | Observations about patient |
|---|---|
| 1 | No pain. Relaxed, freely moving. Does not notice surgical site palpation. Normal attention to environment. Interactive, playful. Normal physiologic parameters. |
| 2 | Slightly painful. Carries head and neck almost normally. Looks at surgical site when palpated (orients to surgical site), but does not resent it. Attentive, avoids interaction. |
| 3 | Mildly painful. Restricted movement. Orients to site, objects to palpation of the surgical site. Somewhat restless. |
| 4 | Moderately painful. Marked guarding of surgical site, neck extended. Tries to escape palpation of the surgical site. May bite. Limited interest in surroundings. Restless, vocalizes, responds to comforting. |
| 5 | Very painful. Pain could not be worse. Tense, shivering, rigid. Avoids touch, may bite, paws at bandage. Unsolicited vocalization. May have very shallow, labored breathing; increased heart rate; and fixed stare. May not move at all. |

Note: If a behavior is normally present, do not include it in your scoring. For example, if a dog bites you in the exam that assesses its temperament, you cannot use biting to evaluate analgesia.

***Table 5-2.*** *Scoring system used to evaluate analgesia in cats after an onychectomy (unpublished data).*

| Analgesia score | Observations about patient |
|---|---|
| 1 | No pain. Relaxed, freely moving. Does not resent palpation of the surgical site. Normal attention to environment. Playfully interactive. Normal physiologic parameters. |
| 2 | Faintly painful. Barely noticeable alteration from normal. May have slightly abnormal stance or gait. Looks at surgical site during palpation (orients to palpation site), but does not resent it. Observant, but restricted interaction. May sit with one paw raised, but stands on all paws. |
| 3 | Mildly painful. Slightly restricted movement. Holds one paw raised. May stand slightly arched or tucked, with toes just touching the floor. Orients and withdraws from palpation site. Licks paws. |
| 4 | Moderately painful. Noticeably arched, abnormal posture. Non-weight bearing. Tries to escape palpation. May bite. Marked guarding. May chew, bite, or shake foot. May cry or growl. Limited interest in surroundings. Will move around, and may be restless. |
| 5 | Very painful. Pain could not be worse. Tense, writhing, shivering, shuddering. May not move at all. May be rigid. Non-weight bearing. May refuse to walk or stand. May be self-mutilating. May have fixed stare. Unsolicited crying, growling. May have very shallow, labored breathing and increased heart rate. |

Note: If a behavior is normally present, do not include it in your scoring. For example, if a cat bites you in the exam that assesses its temperament, you cannot use biting to evaluate analgesia.

***Figure 5-1****. Attributes that owners were able to distinguish in post-onychectomy cats (unpublished observation). Owners assigned scores for each attribute on the first and second days at home after their pets had an onychectomy.*

**Appetite:** Please score your cat's appetite for the first day home as follows:

1: ________ Ate more than normal.

2: ________ Ate about the normal amount.

3: ________ Ate about the normal amount, with coaxing.

4: ________ Ate less than the normal amount, but did eat something. This would include a cat that ate different food than normal.

5: ________ Did not eat at all.

**Personality/Demeanor:** Please score your cat's personality for the first day home as follows:

1: ________ More aggressive or restless than normal.

2: ________ About normal.

3: ________ Slightly less active than normal, but seems to be feeling normal.

4: ________ Less active than normal and somewhat depressed.

5: ________ Depressed, unresponsive, hides, avoids contact.

**Gait (Lameness) Score:** Please score your cat's gait for the first day home as follows:

1: ________ Sound. Walks, runs, and plays normally.

2: ________ Slightly uncomfortable when walking or playing. Barely noticeable. May shift weight from one foot to the other when standing or sitting. Not lame if running.

3: ________ Noticeable lameness, but weight bearing. Places foot down when standing. Does walk on both feet.

4: ________ Bears weight occasionally, especially if needed for balance, but tends not to walk or run. At rest, holds one or both feet up.

5: ________ Non–weight bearing. Will not walk, stand, or run if it can avoid doing so.

chemicals, so it is difficult to interpret the results. Many factors in addition to pain can affect the concentrations of the hormones and metabolites in blood (e.g., drugs, surgery, stress, anesthesia); they cannot be used to differentiate between inadequate pain management and environmental stress. Therefore, they are not very specific. Conzemius et al.[4] has suggested that if the degree of stress in an animal could be decreased, blood concentrations of cortisol, epinephrine, and norepinephrine might be more meaningful. It is critical to collect and handle the samples properly for stress-related hormone and metabolite assays; time intervals for sample collections are not well established. Although these variables are valuable in research settings, at present, they have limited clinical usefulness for an individual. Continued research may increase the value of these variables as objective measures of pain and analgesia.

When evaluating a patient, consider the dose of analgesic that has been administered, the analgesic's duration of action, and how much time has lapsed since administering the analgesic. The response to palpation of a surgical wound, the response to abdominal palpation, the degree of lameness, and the extent to which a patient guards a limb or an injury may be assessed serially to detect increased comfort. Analgesics should not be withheld so that the remission of pain can be used to determine the success of the surgery or the progression of the disease. Consistent and thorough evaluations of the patient should be used to determine the success of the surgery, the progression of the disease, and the effectiveness of the analgesic protocol.

## References

1. Smith JD, Allen SW, Quandt JE, Tackett RL. Indicators of postoperative pain in cats. Am J Vet Res 1996; 57:1674–8.
2. Hellyer PW, Gaynor JS. Acute postsurgical pain in dogs and cats. Compendium Continuing Educ Practicing Vet 1998; 20:140–53.
3. Holton LL, Scott EM, Nolan AM, Reid J, Welsh E, Flaherty D. Comparison of three methods for assessment of pain in dogs. J Am Vet Med Assoc 1998; 212:61–6.
4. Conzemius MG, Hill CM, Sammarco JL, Perkowski SZ. Correlation between subjective and objective measures used to determine severity of postoperative pain in dogs. J Am Vet Med Assoc 1997; 210:1619–22.
5. Buback JL, Boothe HW, Carroll GL, Green RW. Comparison of three methods for relief of pain after ear canal ablation in dogs. Vet Surg 1996; 25:380–5.
6. Hardie EM, Hansen BD, Carroll GS. Behavior after ovariohysterectomy in the dog: what's normal? Appl Anim Behav 1997; 51:111–28.

# Chapter 6 Sample Cases

In this chapter, anesthetic and analgesic regimens will be described for surgical and medical management of painful small animal veterinary patients. These regimens are only suggestions; an individual patient may respond to treatment differently, thereby requiring an adjustment of dose, route, dosing interval, or drug compared to the patient in the example. Some of the cases illustrate that several treatment options are available for a given condition. In all cases, the treatment that the veterinarian chooses should be consistent with the level of discomfort that the patient is experiencing.

## Acute Trauma-Analgesia When Stabilizing the Patient

Analgesia for patients that have been acutely traumatized is important since pain can contribute to deterioration of their status. In all cases of acute trauma, appropriate measures should be taken to stabilize the patient. Generally, these patients require blood-volume replacement (e.g., crystalloids, colloids, hypertonic saline, blood products). Life-threatening injuries should be addressed (e.g., airway and ventilation, penetrating chest wounds, uncontrolled hemorrhage). Oxygen may be supplemented by face mask or nasal insufflation. Drugs with profound cardiopulmonary side effects should either not be administered during this time or the dosage of these drugs should be carefully titrated to effect and the patient monitored closely for decompensation.

## Case No. 1 — Canine with a Pelvis Fracture That Was Hit by a Car

*Signalment*

A 32-kg, 2-year-old intact male German Shepherd is presented after being hit by a car. The dog is recumbent but responsive.

*Physical Exam*

The patient has pale mucous membranes (mm) with a CRT of 3 seconds. PCV = 35%, TS = 6.0 gm/dl. Heart rate (HR) is 170 beats per minute (bpm); respiratory rate (RR) is 60 breaths per minute (rpm); body temperature (T) is 37.2°C (99°F). Thorax is normal on auscultation and abdominal palpation is unremarkable; bladder is palpable.

*Perioperative Care*

A cephalic IV catheter is placed and crystalloids are administered at 90 ml/kg/hr for 15 minutes, and the patient's status is reassessed. Mucous membranes are pink; CRT is <2 seconds. Intravenous fluids are slowed to a maintenance rate (30 ml/kg/day). Thoracic and abdominal radiographs are within normal limits, but the pelvis is fractured. The dog is scheduled for surgery the following day. An area over the dorsal cervical spine is clipped and a 100-μg/hr fentanyl patch is placed. Since the fentanyl patch will not be effective for at least 12 hours, additional analgesics may be necessary for pain associated with the trauma. The patient is monitored for signs of decompensation. The next day, HR = 90 bpm, RR = 24 rpm, T = 38.3°C (101°F), mm = pink, CRT <2 seconds. PCV = 32%, TS = 5.5 gm/dl,
BUN = 16 mg/dl; urine has been voided during the night. The thorax is normal on auscultation and the abdominal palpation is normal. A rhythm strip (ECG, lead II) indicates no arrhythmias.

*Anesthetic Protocol*

**Premedicant**: glycopyrrolate (0.011 mg/kg, SC). If sedation is inadequate preoperatively, oxymorphone (0.05 mg/kg, IM) may be administered with the anticholinergic. Preoxygenation may be beneficial.
**Induction**: thiopental (12 mg/kg, IV) or propofol (4 mg/kg, IV) to effect.
**Maintenance**: isoflurane or sevoflurane in oxygen; the fentanyl patch (see Figure 6-1) contributes to intraoperative analgesia. At recovery, breakthrough pain may be treated with fentanyl (0.002 to 0.005 mg/kg, IV) or oxymorphone (0.05 to 0.1 mg/kg, IV). Dysphoria may be treated with acepromazine (0.05 mg/kg, IV, not to

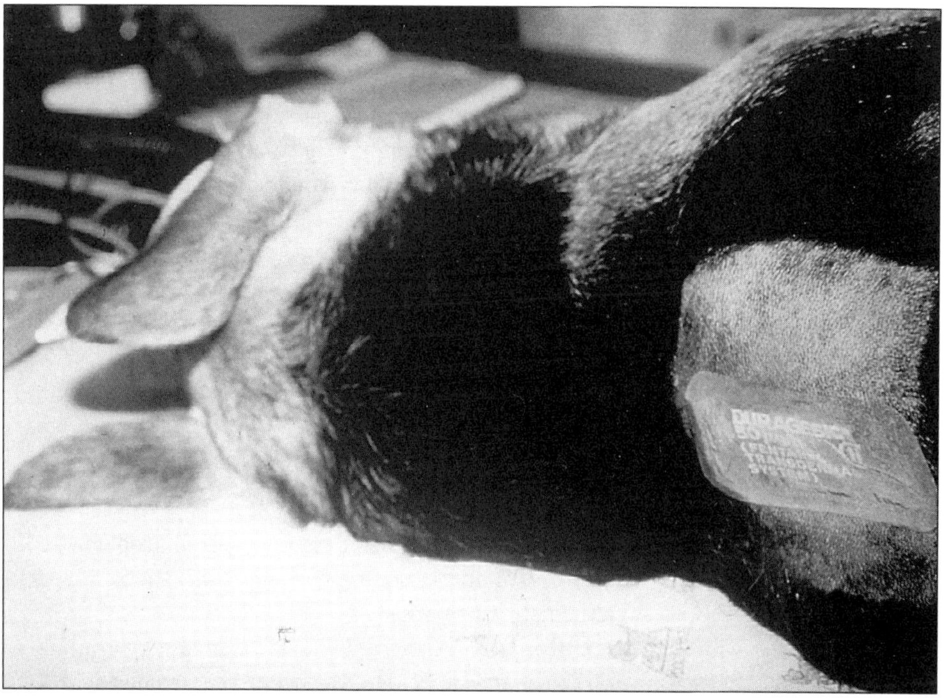

*Figure 6-1. A 100-µg/hour fentanyl patch in place for surgery. The patch was placed the day before surgery. Note the patch should be protected from external heat sources.*

exceed 1 mg, diluted in 10 ml of sterile water) titrated to effect. The fentanyl patch should be removed 72 hours after placement; the patch may be replaced if necessary.

*Alternative Analgesic Therapy*

An alternative treatment for this dog would be to manage the acute pain with buprenorphine for the first day and perform an opioid epidural (oxymorphone, morphine, or buprenorphine) the following day after anesthetic induction and prior to surgery. Although buprenorphine does not appear as efficacious for moderate to severe pain as pure µ-agonists, it should produce less sedation and cardiopulmonary side effects than a pure µ-agonist; this might be advantageous in a recently traumatized patient if cardiopulmonary function is compromised significantly.

## Case No. 2 — Feline Fan-Belt Injury

*Signalment*

A 2-year-old female DSH cat weighing 6 kg is presented for skin wounds believed to have occurred about 4 hours earlier. The patient was not fed that morning.

*Physical Exam*

On physical exam, the patient is bright and alert with stable cardiopulmonary function. HR = 140 bpm, RR = purring, T = 37.7°C (100°F), mm = pink, CRT = <2 seconds. The patient has several small lacerations over the torso, a degloving injury to right forelimb, and a large (4-cm) semicircular wound covering the right hip. PCV = 29%, TS = 5.4 gm/dl, BUN = 5 to 15 mg/dl (stick method).

*Perioperative Care*

Immediate surgery is planned to clean and suture the wounds. A cephalic IV catheter is placed and a balanced electrolyte solution is administered IV; a broad-spectrum antibiotic is administered.

*Anesthetic Protocol*

**Premedicants**: glycopyrrolate (0.011 mg/kg, IM) and buprenorphine (0.015 mg/kg, IM).
**Induction**: Anesthesia is induced with diazepam (0.27 mg/kg, IV) and ketamine (5.5 mg/kg, IV) mixed, and administered to effect.
**Maintenance**: Anesthesia is maintained with isoflurane or halothane in oxygen. Recovery and analgesia are monitored postoperatively. Buprenorphine (0.015 mg/kg, IM) is administered 6 hours after the original dose and every 8 hours thereafter for 48 hours.

*Alternative Analgesic Therapy*

An alternative for this patient would be to apply a fentanyl patch (25 μg/hour), particularly if primary closure of the wounds is impossible, and analgesia is expected to be necessary for at least 3 days.

---

## Surgical Cases

### Case No. 3 — Elective Surgery: Feline Onychectomy

*Signalment*

A 5-month-old castrated male DSH cat weighing 3 kg is presented for an onychectomy.

*Physical Exam*

The physical exam is normal. PCV = 37%, TS = 6.8 gm/dl.

*Anesthetic Protocol*

**Premedicants**: butorphanol (0.4 mg/kg, SC or IM); acepromazine (0.025 mg/kg, SC or IM; reduced dosages of acepromazine are used in cats younger than 6 months); glycopyrrolate (0.011 mg/kg, SC, IM); ketamine (10 mg/kg, IM). The premedicants can be mixed and administered IM.

**Induction**: mask induction with halothane or isoflurane in oxygen, although isoflurane is preferred for mask or chamber inductions.
**Maintenance**: halothane or isoflurane in oxygen.
**Intraoperative bupivacaine**: One drop per toe of 0.5% bupivacaine delivered from a tuberculin syringe without a needle may be administered prior to bandaging. Do not exceed 1 mg/kg total dose of bupivacaine; generally, 0.25 ml of 0.5% bupivacaine (1.25 mg) divided among 10 toes (one drop per toe) can be used for kittens as small as 1.4 kg. A second injection of butorphanol (0.4 mg/kg, SC, IM) should be administered 4 to 6 hours after the first dose. The next morning, the cat can be started on oral butorphanol (0.4 mg/kg [$\frac{1}{2}$ of a 5-mg or $\frac{1}{4}$ of a 10-mg tablet]; generally, not to exceed 1 mg/kg). Oral butorphanol should be administered three times daily for 2 days. The butorphanol may be dispensed to the owner if the cat is discharged before the end of the 2 days, with instructions to confine the cat and to observe the cat for sedation.

## Case No. 4 — Elective Surgery: Canine Ovariohysterectomy (OVH)

*Signalment*

An 8-month-old female Labrador Retriever weighing 29 kg is presented for an ovariohysterectomy.

*Physical Exam*

The physical exam is normal. PCV = 35%, TS = 7.0 gm/dl.

*Anesthetic Protocol*

**Premedicants**: buprenorphine (0.015 mg/kg, IM); acepromazine (0.05 mg/kg, SC or IM, not to exceed 1 mg); glycopyrrolate (0.011 mg/kg, SC or IM).
**Induction**: thiopental (12 mg/kg, IV to effect).
**Maintenance**: halothane or isoflurane in oxygen. Buprenorphine (0.015 mg/kg, IM) may be redosed 6 hours after the original dose. Clinically, the IM route of buprenorphine administration appears to provide better results than the SC route of administration. A small needle (e.g., 23 gauge) is recommended for all IM injections.

*Alternative Analgesic Therapy*

Butorphanol (0.4 mg/kg, SC or IM) could be substituted for the buprenorphine, but the redosing schedule would be more frequent (every 3 to 4 hours for at least two postoperative treatments). Morphine (0.4 mg/kg, IM or SC) would be an inexpensive alternative to butorphanol or buprenorphine.

## Case No. 5 — Orthopedic Surgery: Feline Bilateral Femoral Head Fractures

*Signalment*

A 1-year-old male castrated DSH cat weighing 5.5 kg is presented with a 2-week history of bilateral hindlimb lameness. The patient is currently on a decreasing oral dosage of steroids for allergic dermatitis.

*Physical Exam*

The physical exam (except for musculoskeletal) is normal. Pain is elicited during palpation of the hips; the patellas luxate easily.

*Perioperative Care*

The patient was administered glycopyrrolate (0.011 mg/kg, IM) and butorphanol (0.2 mg/kg, IM) followed 25 minutes later by medetomidine (total dose = 0.25 ml [0.25 mg], IV) for pelvic radiographs. Radiographs indicated bilateral femoral head fractures. Atipamezole (total dose = 0.25 ml [1.25 mg], IM) was administered to antagonize medetomidine. Surgery was scheduled for the next day. Since 6 to 12 hours are needed for fentanyl plasma concentrations to plateau, a site was prepared for a transdermal fentanyl patch to be placed in preparation for surgery the next day. The fur was clipped over the dorsal cervical spine and a 25-µg/hr fentanyl patch was placed. The cat was discharged in the care of its owner, a veterinarian. The owner called 3 hours later to say that the cat continued to rub against furniture in an attempt to remove the patch. The owner could not confine the cat and feared that the cat would aggravate his preexisting injury. The owner was advised to remove the patch, fold it on itself, and return it to the hospital the next day. Although fentanyl patches have been placed successfully on many cats, in retrospect this cat was not a good candidate for patch placement. The owner wished to have the cat at home and the cat was not disabled by his injury, so he could dedicate himself to removal of the patch. This has not been a problem in painful hospitalized cats. A less desirable alternative to patch removal would have been to tranquilize the cat with acepromazine for the evening. The cat was fasted and presented for surgery the next day. Since this regimen was unsuccessful, the anesthetic protocol was altered.

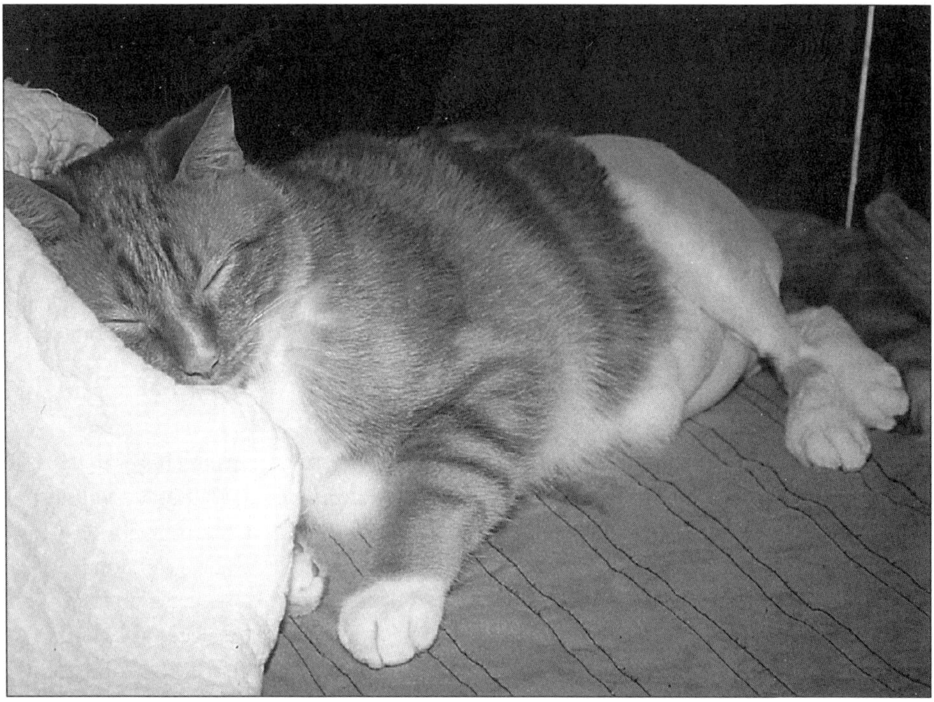

***Figure 6-2***. *This cat rested comfortably after bilateral hip surgery. A morphine epidural was used for analgesia.*

*Anesthetic Protocol*

**Premedicants**: ketamine (5 mg/kg, IM) and glycopyrrolate (0.011 mg/kg, IM).
**Induction**: propofol (4 mg/kg, IV to effect).
**Maintenance**: isoflurane or sevoflurane in oxygen. An epidural is planned using preservative-free morphine (Duramorph 0.1 mg/kg); due to the extension of the dural sac in cats, a spinal is accomplished; see Appendix A for an explanation of this technique. The right femoral head and neck is resected; the left femoral head is reduced and screwed. The surgery lasts approximately 4.5 hours. At recovery, the cat appears slightly dysphoric, but is not believed to be painful since he attempts to stand on his operated legs. Acepromazine (0.025 mg/kg, IV) is administered. The cat rests comfortably (see Figure 6-2) until the next morning when oral butorphanol ($^1/_2$ of a 5-mg tablet, PO TID) is administered. The following day, the cat is discharged with oral butorphanol to be administered at the discretion of the owner, a veterinarian. The oral butorphanol was used twice daily for 2 days.

## Case No. 6 Orthopedic Surgery: Canine Forelimb Amputation

*Signalment*

A 9-year-old, 47-kg Rottweiler is presented for forelimb lameness. The dog has received carprofen (100 mg twice daily, orally) for 7 days.

*Physical Exam*

The physical exam is unremarkable except for a painful swelling of the proximal humerus. Radiographs and biopsy results are consistent with osteosarcoma. Thoracic radiographs show no evidence of metastasis. Screening blood work is within normal limits. Amputation is recommended and surgery is scheduled for the next day.

*Perioperative Care*

Precautions which may be taken during this surgery include IV fluids to maintain circulating blood volume and renal blood flow, appropriate hemostasis to decrease blood loss and hypovolemia, and minimum vaporizer settings to guard against reduced cardiac output, hypotension, and compromised renal blood flow. Serial measurements of hematocrit and total solids are indicated if hemorrhage becomes extensive. Since this patient has received NSAIDs, maintenance of normal blood pressure is important to assure blood flow. Drugs that promote hypotension and interfere with platelet function (e.g., acepromazine) should be avoided preoperatively.

*Anesthetic Protocol*

**Premedicants**: oxymorphone (0.1 mg/kg, IM) and glycopyrrolate (0.011 mg/kg, IM).
**Induction**: thiopental (12 mg/kg, IV) or propofol (4 mg/kg, IV) to effect. Maintenance on isoflurane or sevoflurane in oxygen. Brachial plexus block is performed with bupivacaine (total maximum dose is 2 mg/kg; use up to 1 mg/kg for the preoperative regional nerve block and inject up to 1 mg/kg of bupivacaine directly into nerve stump during surgery). Surgery requires 2 hours. At extubation, oxymorphone (0.05 mg/kg, IV) is administered. Oxymorphone may be redosed (IM, SC, or IV) at 4- to 6-hour intervals.

*Alternative Analgesic Therapy*

There are other alternatives for managing pain associated with forelimb amputations. Injectable morphine may be used systemically instead of oxymorphone, but morphine should not be administered as a bolus intravenously. A morphine epidural may be administered (see thoracotomy case, Case No. 8) after anesthetic induction. Another option is a fentanyl patch, applied preoperatively (12 to 24 hours), with breakthrough pain treated as needed using fentanyl, oxymorphone, or morphine.

## Case No. 7 — Orthopedic Surgery: Canine Cranial Cruciate Rupture

*Signalment*

A 2-year-old male Golden Retriever weighing 36 kg is presented for lameness of the right hindlimb.

*Physical Exam*

The physical exam is normal, except for the ruptured right cranial cruciate ligament.

*Anesthetic Protocol*

**Premedicants**: glycopyrrolate (0.011 mg/kg, SC, IM) and morphine (0.4 mg/kg, IM or SC).
**Induction**: thiopental (12 mg/kg, IV) or propofol (4 mg/kg, IV) to effect.
**Maintenance**: isoflurane or halothane. Intraoperatively, intra-articular bupivacaine (up to 2 mg/kg) is administered after joint closure. Morphine (0.4 mg/kg, IM or SC) may be administered 4 hours after the original dose. The patient may be discharged on carprofen (2.2 mg/kg, PO BID).

*Analgesic Alternatives*

There are several alternatives for analgesia in this dog. The type of repair performed (intracapsular, extracapsular) and the amount of preexisting degenerative joint disease contribute to the amount of postoperative pain. Systemic buprenorphine or butorphanol may be sufficient for dogs undergoing minimally invasive surgery (mild to moderate pain). Alternatively, intra-articular morphine (0.1 mg/kg diluted with saline to a volume of 0.5 ml/kg) may be used for analgesia instead of bupivacaine.

## Case No. 8 — Soft-Tissue Surgery: Canine Thoracotomy

*Signalment*

A 7-year-old female Labrador Retriever weighing 24 kg is presented with pyothorax.

*Physical Exam*

The physical exam reveals a well-nourished dog with muffled lung sounds in all fields. The patient is nervous. Mucous membranes become slightly cyanotic with struggling. Pyothorax is confirmed by cytology of thoracic fluid. The patient is scheduled for a thoracotomy (median sternotomy) the next day. Blood screening tests indicate: PCV = 28.5%, TS = 8.2 gm/dl and a leucocytosis (30.2 x $10^3/\mu l$) with a mature neutrophilia (20.8 x $10^3/\mu l$) and a monocytosis (4.8 x $10^3/\mu l$).

*Anesthetic Protocol*

**Premedicants**: acepromazine (0.05 mg/kg, IM not to exceed 1 mg) and glycopyrrolate (0.011 mg/kg, IM). The dog is observed after premedication and is oxygenated by mask during IV catheter placement and induction.
**Induction**: thiopental (12 mg/kg, IV) or propofol (4 mg/kg, IV) to effect.
**Maintenance**: isoflurane or sevoflurane in oxygen; intermittent positive pressure ventilation at 8 breaths per minute and 20 cm of $H_2O$ inspiratory pressure. A preservative-free morphine epidural (Duramorph 0.1 mg/kg) is administered after induction. Bilateral thoracic drains are placed during surgery. The thorax is closed and negative pressure is achieved. Bupivacaine (2 mg/kg) is diluted to a volume of 20 ml and half is instilled through each thoracic drain. The dog is placed on its sternum for 20 minutes after administration of bupivacaine. The chest is wrapped and a nasal cannula (e.g., red rubber feeding tube) is inserted through one nostril and into the nasopharynx and secured for insufflation of oxygen. Pulse oximetry is used to evaluate oxygenation during recovery. The inhalant is discontinued once the patient is ventilating normally, and the patient is extubated (see Figure 6-3). The oxygen saturation of this patient is 96% postoperatively. HR (117 bpm) and RR (14 rpm) are normal. Oxymorphone (0.05 to 0.1 mg/kg, IV) could be used to treat breakthrough pain if necessary. This patient rests comfortably through the night.

## Case No. 9 — Soft-Tissue Surgery: Feline Thyroidectomy

*Signalment*

A 13-year-old, 4-kg DSH cat is diagnosed with hyperthyroidism. Current medications include propranolol (β-blocker) and methimazole (Tapazole, an antithyroid).

*Physical Exam*

The physical exam reveals a palpable thyroid gland. The patient is thin. The HR is 190 bpm, the RR is 36, and the body temperature is 38.9°C (102°F). The ECG is consistent with ventricular thickening seen with hyperthyroidism.

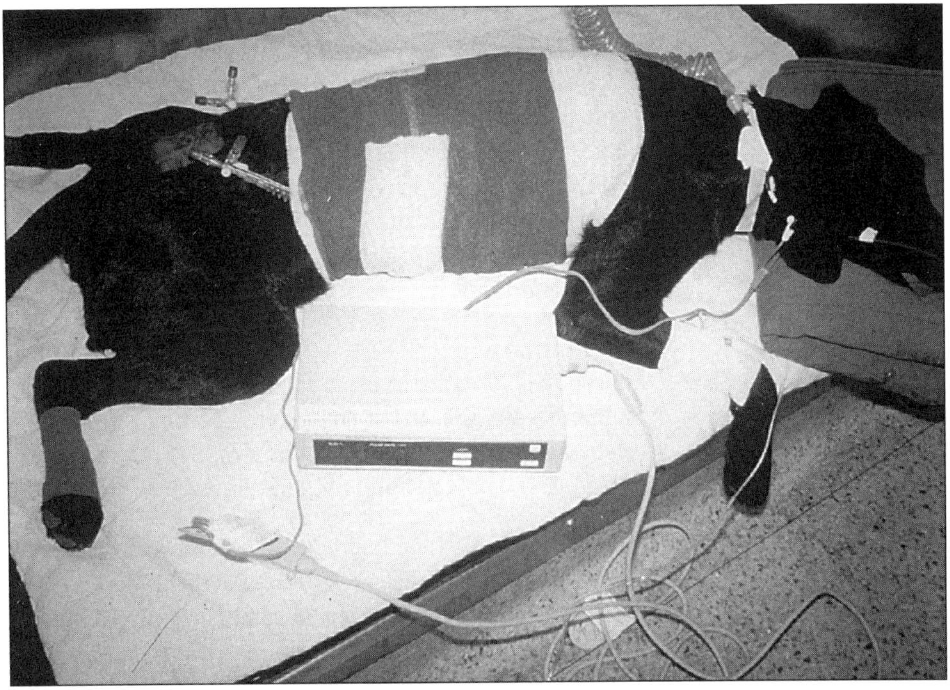

*Figure 6-3. This dog rested comfortably after a sternotomy. A morphine epidural and interpleural bupivacaine were used for analgesia. The patient's oxygen saturation is acceptable (96%) and the heart rate is normal. (Photograph courtesy of Dr. Elizabeth Martinez.)*

*Anesthetic Protocol*

**Premedication**: butorphanol (0.4 mg/kg, IM).
**Induction**: diazepam (0.2 mg/kg, IV) followed immediately by etomidate (2 mg/kg, IV to effect).
**Maintenance**: isoflurane or sevoflurane in oxygen.
Precautions during surgery: continuous ECG monitoring; arterial blood pressure monitoring. Surgery requires 1.5 hours. At extubation, HR is elevated (250 bpm) and the cat appears anxious. Butorphanol (0.2 mg/kg, IV) is administered and the patient rests comfortably. Four to 6 hours after the second dose of butorphanol, an additional dose (butorphanol 0.4 mg/kg, SC) may be administered.

## Medical Cases

### Case No. 10 — Canine Pancreatitis

*Signalment*

An 8-year-old spayed female miniature poodle (7.5 kg) is presented with vomiting and a painful abdomen. The dog ingested sausage the previous day.

*Physical Exam*

The physical exam reveals a depressed dog with a painful abdomen, "muddy" mucous membranes, and a CRT of 3 seconds. The dog is estimated to be 10% dehydrated. The HR is 160 bpm and the dog is panting; body temperature is 39.4°C (103°F). Screening blood work reveals elevated amylase and lipase values. The dog is hospitalized and closely monitored. Although the patient is depressed, she does not appear to be able to get comfortable and has a glazed appearance in her eyes.

*Treatment Plan*

A cephalic IV catheter is placed and the patient is administered a balanced electrolyte solution to correct dehydration. Butorphanol (0.4 mg/kg, SC) is administered. The dog is not allowed food or water.

*Patient Reassessment*

The patient's attitude improves; she becomes interested in her surroundings. Her HR decreases to 110 beats per minute, and RR decreases to 16 rpm. Mucous membrane color and refill time improve. Fluids are continued and butorphanol is administered every 4 to 6 hours for about 24 hours.

## Case No. 11 — Feline Cancer Patient

*Signalment*

An 11-year-old Siamese spayed female cat weighing 3 kg is diagnosed with nonresectable oral squamous cell carcinoma involving the tongue and mandible. The cat is not eating or grooming. A gastrostomy tube is placed under anesthesia and radiation therapy is begun. The quality of life is believed to be poor due to bone pain. A 25-µg/hr fentanyl patch was placed in the axilla of the cat during the most recent hospitalization; no untoward behavioral or physiologic changes were noted and at the end of 3 days, the patch was removed. The client would like to improve the quality of the cat's life at home. Historically, there is a long-standing and good relationship with this client and cat. The client is retired and will observe the cat closely at home.

*Treatment Plan*

Oral butorphanol ($^1/_4$ to $^1/_2$ a 5-mg tablet, PO TID) can be dispensed. The client is responsible and will reliably administer the butorphanol tablet in food via the gastrostomy tube. There are currently no children or other pets in the household. The client is advised of possible side effects and cautioned to call if there are negative physiologic or behavioral changes. The cat is discharged.

*Alternative Analgesic Therapy*

Another alternative would be to apply a 25-µg/hr fentanyl patch prior to discharge and to have the client return in 3 days for reevaluation. Patients to be discharged with fentanyl patches must be carefully chosen. The legal implications of discharging a patient with a fentanyl patch should be considered. There is the potential for misadventures and abuse; the manufacturer of fentanyl patches discourages their use in veterinary patients. There is the potential for toxicity if a child should come in contact with the patch. If the veterinarian is not comfortable discharging a patient with a fentanyl patch, oral medication is an appropriate alternative. In the case of this cat, as long as oral medication can be administered, butorphanol is an excellent alternative.

# Appendix A Performing Selected Regional Techniques

There are several indications for applying regional techniques. The techniques that are technically simple to perform (e.g., local infiltration, splash blocks, interpleural and intercostal techniques, joint infusions) are described in chapter 3. The two regional techniques included in this appendix require additional supplies and a more detailed description of anatomy than those in chapter 3.

## Technique for Administering Drugs in the Epidural Space

In dogs, neuroleptanalgesia (e.g., glycopyrrolate [0.011 mg/kg, SC, IM] plus butorphanol [0.4 mg/kg, SC, IM] followed in 15 minutes by xylazine [0.2–0.4 mg/kg, IV]) is usually required to safely administer a drug into the epidural space; in cats, general anesthesia is usually required. Supplies needed include a spinal needle, sterile gloves, an appropriate dose and volume of the selected drug, a syringe to administer the drug, a test syringe (3 ml) for air, a 3-ml syringe and a 23-gauge needle for 0.5 to 1 ml of 2% lidocaine for analgesia of the skin in conscious dogs, and a fenestrated drape (eye drape) (see Figure A-1 A). Landmarks for performing epidural technique at $L_7$–$S_1$ intervertebral space are the right and left cranial dorsal iliac spines, the spinous process of $L_7$, and the median sacral crest (see Figures A-1 B and A-1 C). In dogs, the spinal cord variably ends at $L_6$–$L_7$; the dural sac ends at $L_7$–$S_1$. In cats, the cord and sac usually extend one vertebra more caudal (cord termination may be as caudal as $S_3$), so dural punctures are more likely in cats than in dogs.

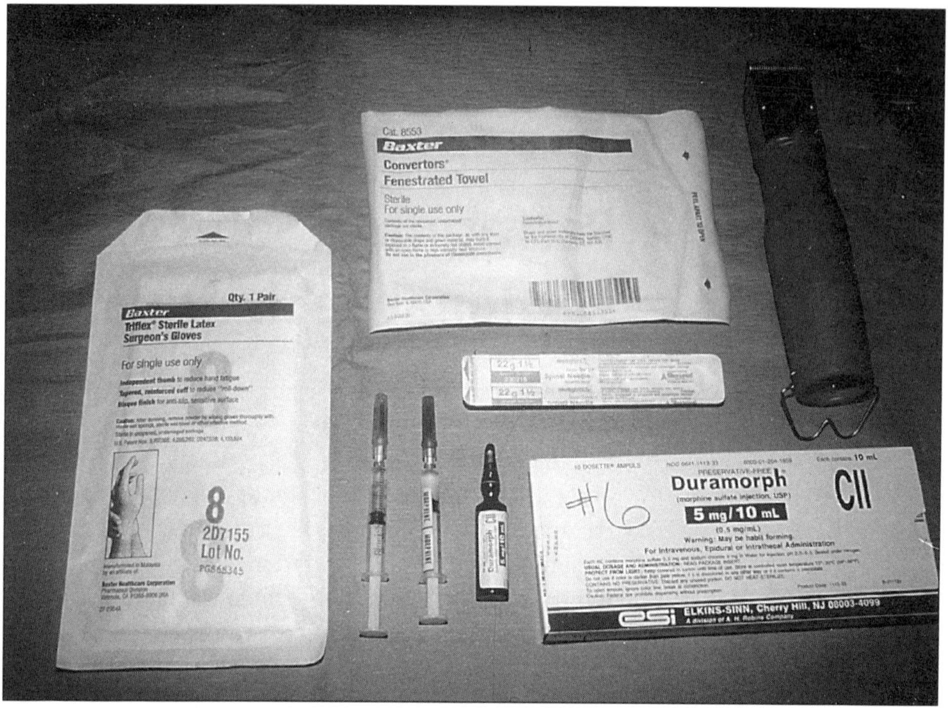


***Figure A-1***. *Performance of a morphine epidural.*
***Figure A-1 A***. *Supplies for performing a morphine epidural: sterile gloves, a fenestrated towel, a spinal needle, preservative-free morphine, a syringe for morphine, and a test syringe with air and/or sterile saline.*

After clipping the area over $L_7$–$S_1$ and performing a sterile preparation, the skin and subcutaneous tissues immediately dorsal to the lumbosacral space are blocked with lidocaine (in the conscious animal). Dogs or cats should be placed in sternal recumbency with the rear limbs flexed and pulled cranially, although the procedure may be performed with the patient in lateral recumbency. Palpate the landmarks; the spinal needle should be inserted through the skin with the bevel craniad (see Figure A-1 D). The notch on the hub of the spinal needle is on the same side as the bevel (see Figure A-1 E). The skin should be penetrated on the dorsal midline perpendicular to the skin in the center of the space between $L_7$ and $S_1$.

An alternate method involves penetrating the skin on the dorsal midline immediately behind and parallel to the spinous process of $L_7$. If one method is unsuccessful, try the other method. Advance the needle through the subcutaneous tissues, the supraspinous ligament,

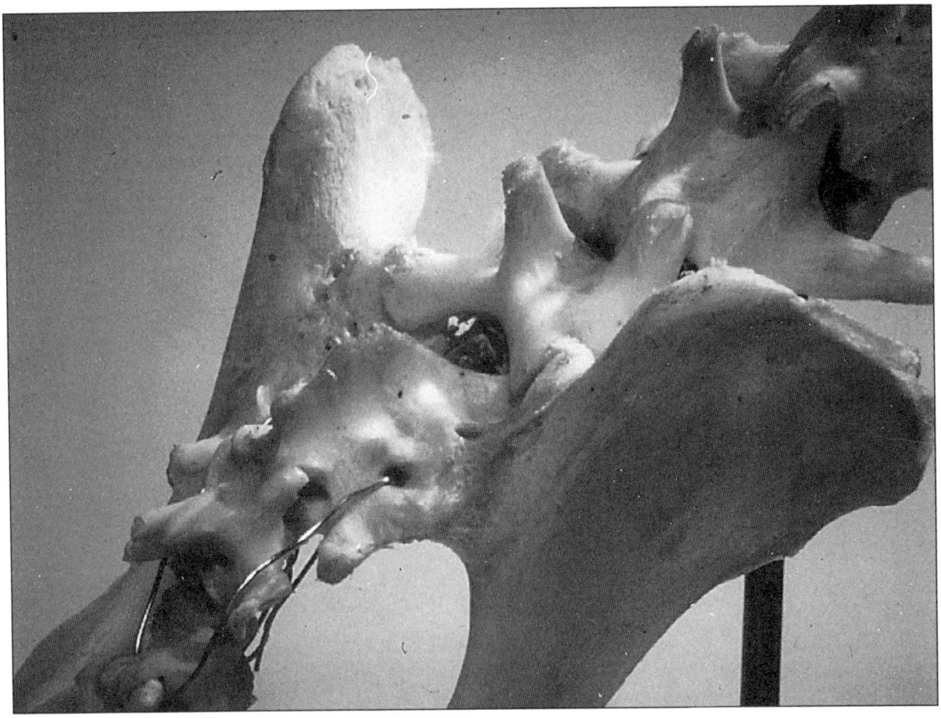

***Figure A-1 B****. Landmarks for performing an epidural in a canine skeleton: wings of the ileum, $L_7$, and the sacral crest.*

the interspinous ligament, and the ligamentum flavum into the epidural space. A "pop" or change in resistance to the advancement of the needle is usually apparent as the ligamentum flavum is penetrated in dogs (not in cats) (see Figure A-1 F). If the spinal needle strikes bone during its advancement, this might mean that the caudal aspect of the spinous process of $L_7$ or the cranial aspect of $S_1$ has been encountered. In that case, withdraw the needle slightly, alter the angle of the needle's penetration cranial or caudal (based on the needle's position in reference to $L_7$ or $S_1$), and gently advance it off the edge of the bone. If proceeding in the craniad direction is unsuccessful, try proceeding in the caudal direction. If neither attempt to enter the space is successful, remove the needle, palpate the landmarks, and try again. To confirm needle placement, remove the stylet and check for spinal fluid or blood (see Figure A-1 G); no spinal fluid should be encountered when an epidural is performed. Gentle aspiration may be performed. If spinal fluid is encountered, the dose of anesthetic should be decreased by half; if blood

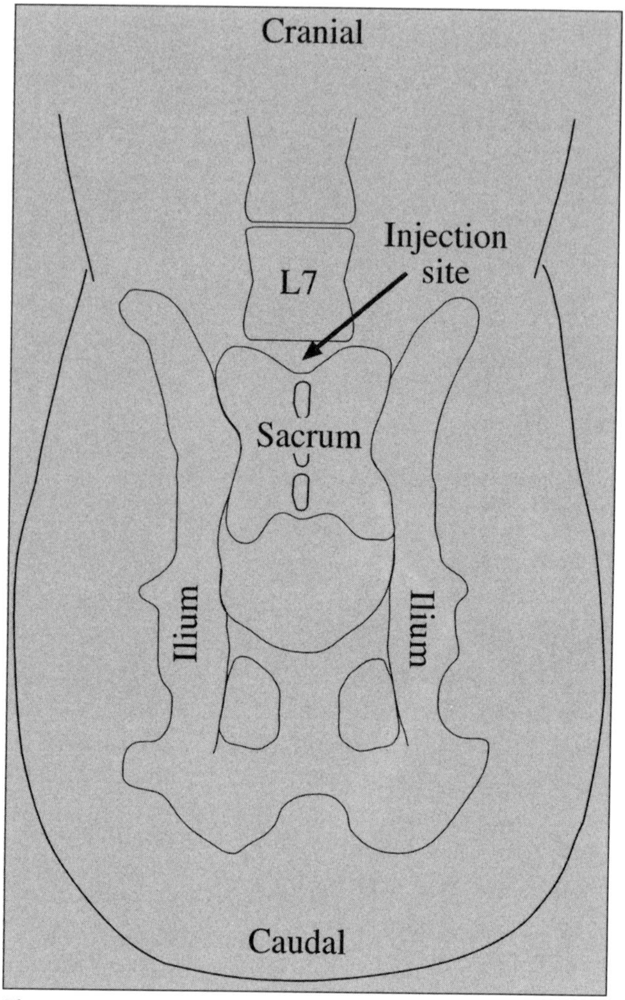


***Figure A-1 C.*** *The dorsal view of a dog with palpable landmarks for epidural injection identified.*

is encountered, the stylet should be replaced and the needle repositioned. Injecting 0.5 ml of air (using 0.5 ml of air and 0.5 ml of saline is acceptable; watch the fluid line for resistance) should not be met with resistance in dogs; use less in cats (0.1 to 0.2 ml of air) (see Figure A-1 H). After the appropriate drug is injected (see Figure A-1 I), replace the stylet (see Figure A-1 J), remove the needle, and position the patient with the affected side (operative site) down. When diluting drugs for use in the epidural space, try to keep the epidural volume below 0.3 ml/kg[1] (or a total volume of 6 ml per dog[1] or 1.5 ml per cat). A similar procedure is followed when placing an epidural cath-

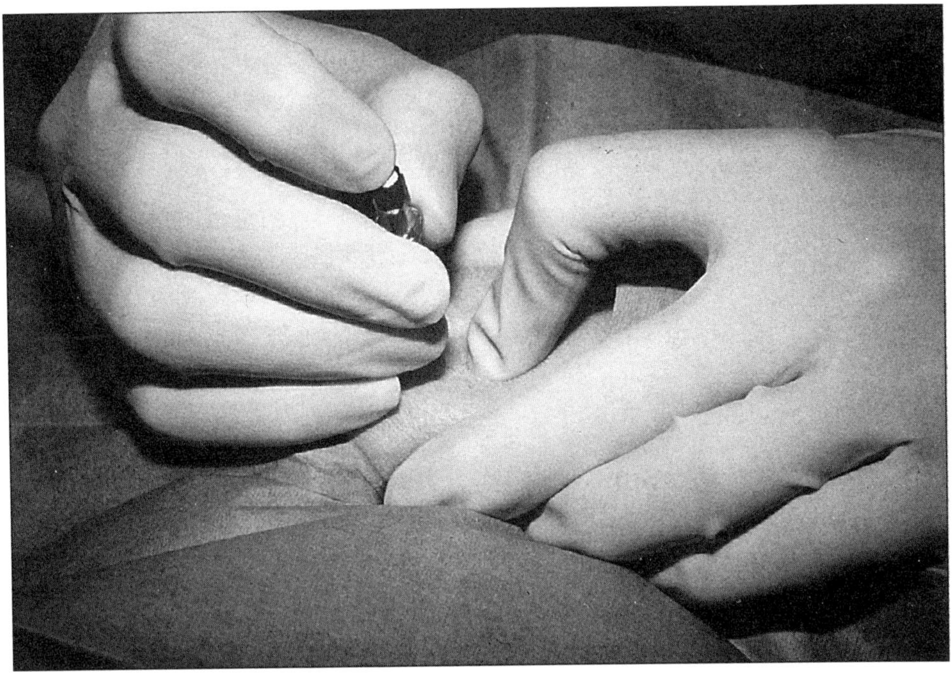

***Figure A-1 D****. After clipping, sterile preparation, and draping, use the nondominant hand to palpate the landmarks; with the dominant hand, enter the skin with the bevel of the spinal needle cranial, perpendicular to the skin, on the dorsal midline.*

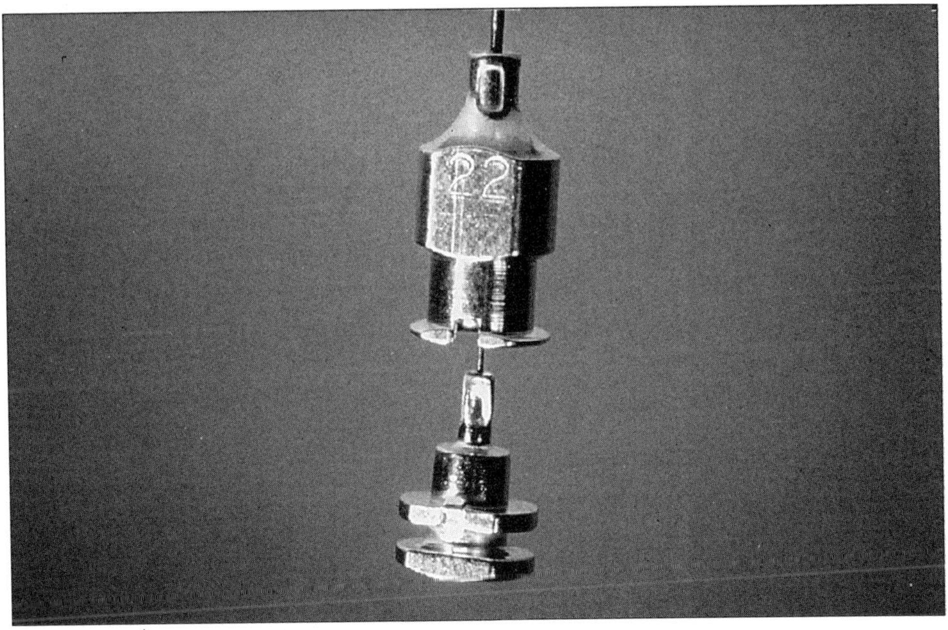


***Figure A-1 E****. Note the notch in a spinal needle. The bevel of the needle is on the same side.*

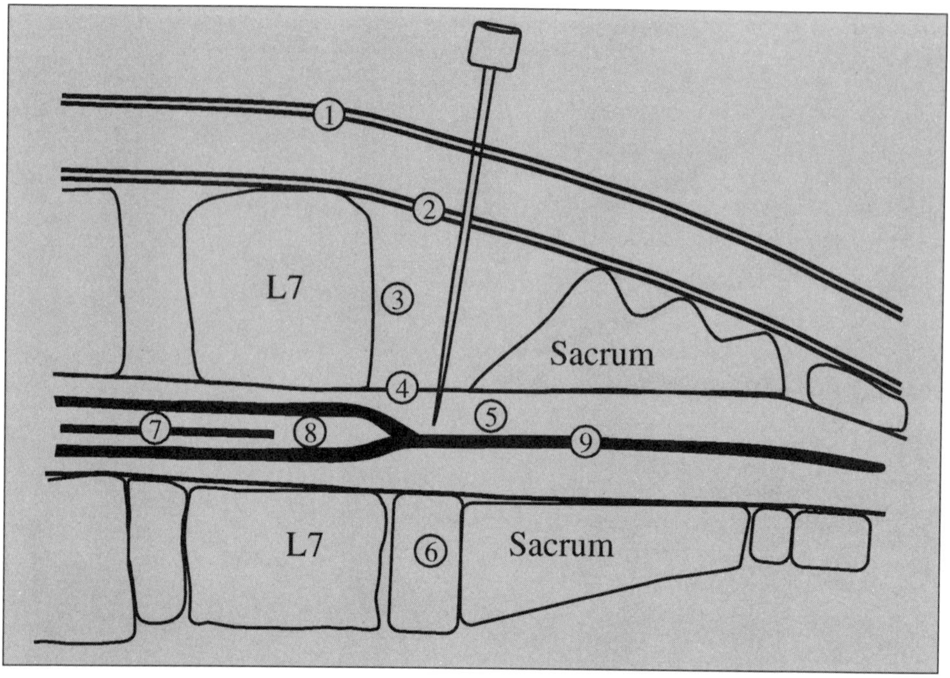


*Figure A-1 F*. The schematic represents the dog's anatomy. 1. skin, 2. supraspinatous ligament, 3. intraspinous ligament, 4. ligamentum flavum, 5. epidural space, 6. intervertebral disc, 7. spinal cord, 8. cerebrospinal fluid, 9. cauda equina. Note the needle placement.

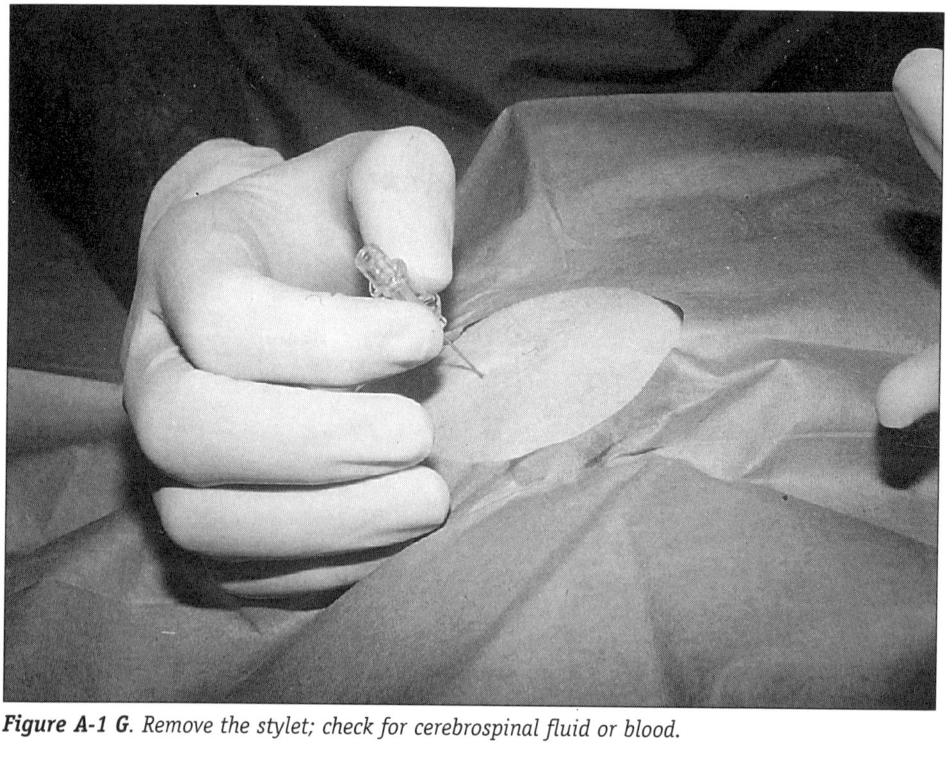

*Figure A-1 G*. Remove the stylet; check for cerebrospinal fluid or blood.

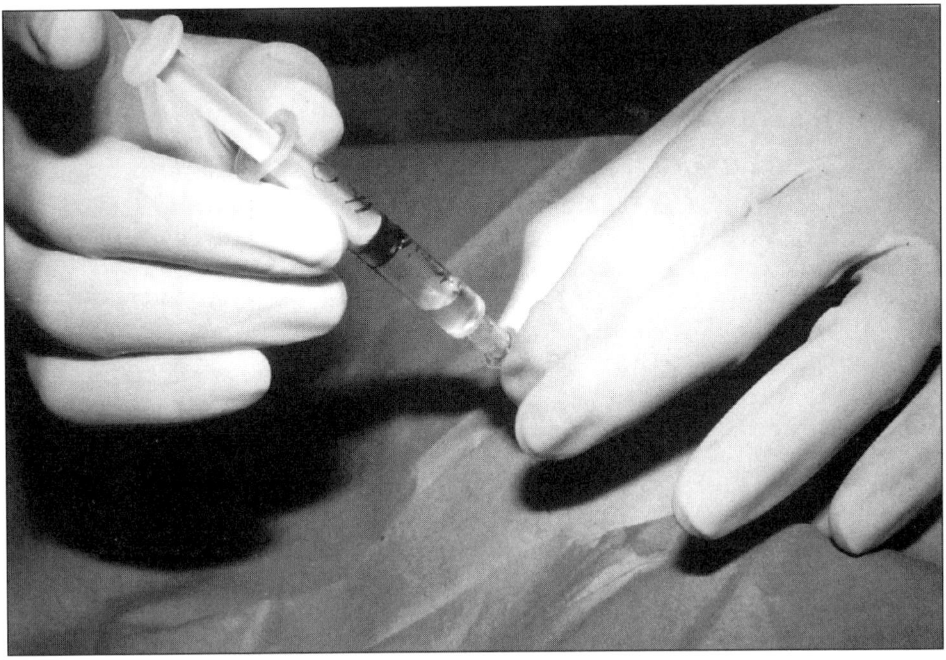

***Figure A-1 H****. A test injection of air, saline, or in this case, air and saline should be made to check for resistance.*

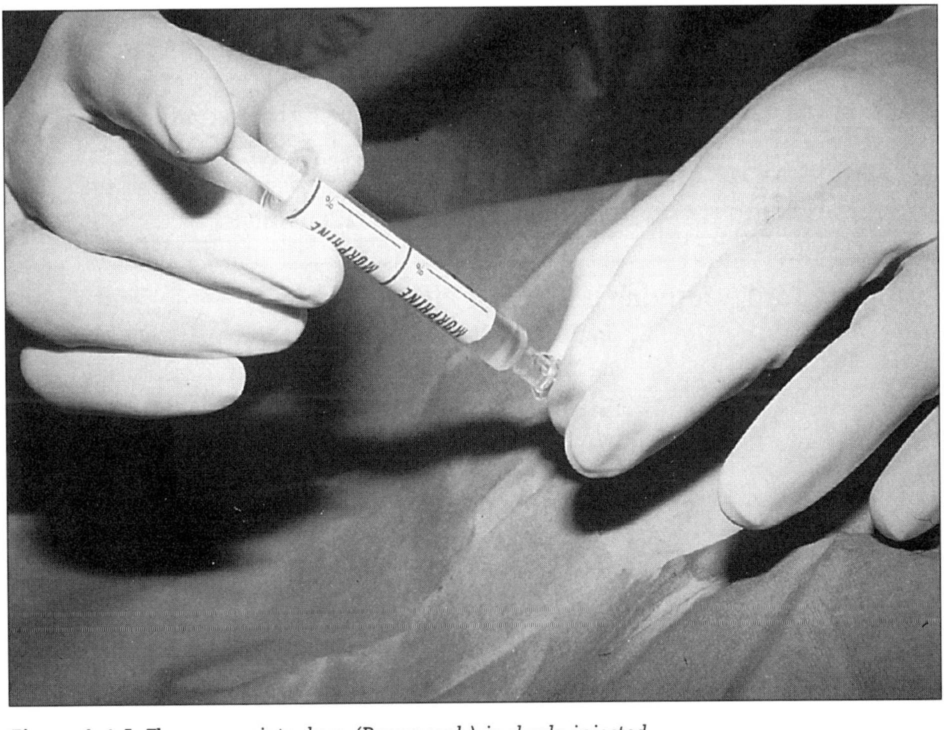


***Figure A-1 I****. The appropriate drug (Duramorph) is slowly injected.*

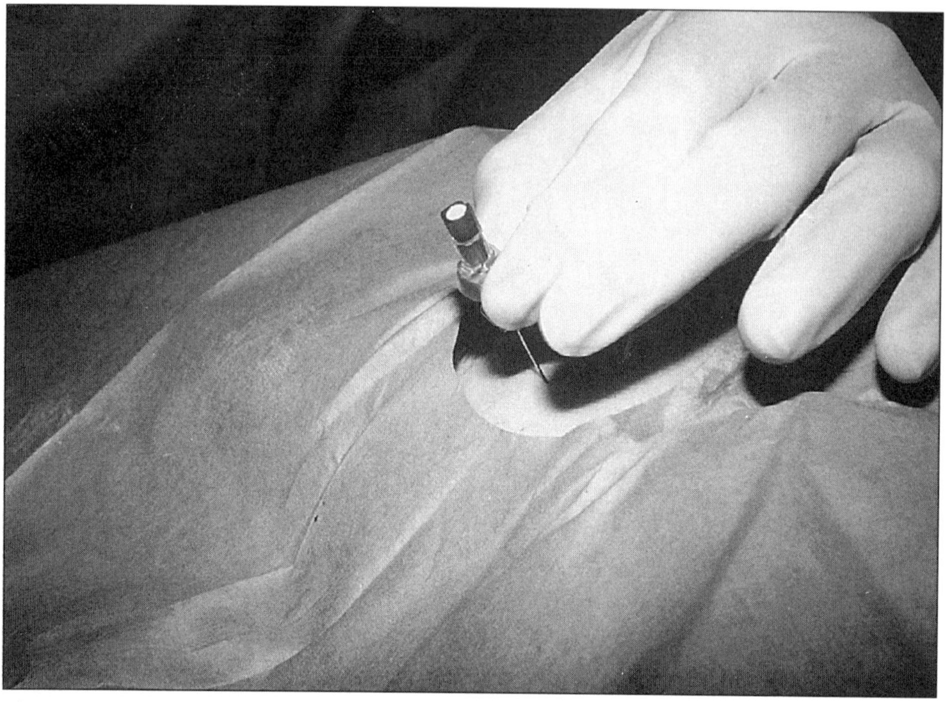

*Figure A-1 J. The stylet is replaced and the needle removed.*

eter; the bevel of a Touhy needle directs the catheter craniad and facilitates catheter placement. Prior to injecting the drug into the catheter, confirm by aspiration that it is placed correctly; doing so will guard against catheter migration and inadvertent intravenous or intrathecal injections.

## Technique for Performing a Brachial Plexus Block

Brachial plexus blocks are most beneficial when they are accomplished preoperatively. After aseptically preparing the site, facilitate the brachial plexus block by inserting a 22-gauge, 3-inch needle (a spinal needle may be used; see Figure A-2 A) in the depression medial to the scapulo-humeral joint and lateral to the thoracic wall, toward the costochondral junction, and parallel to the vertebral column (see Figure A-2 B). Aspirate to assure that the needle is not in a vessel and inject the local anesthetic as the needle is withdrawn (see Figure A-2 C). In cats, a 1.5-inch needle is appropriate for a brachial plexus block. The technique is similar to that for dogs. The needle's depth should be to the middle of the forelimb width at the shoulder joint.[2] Aspirate to

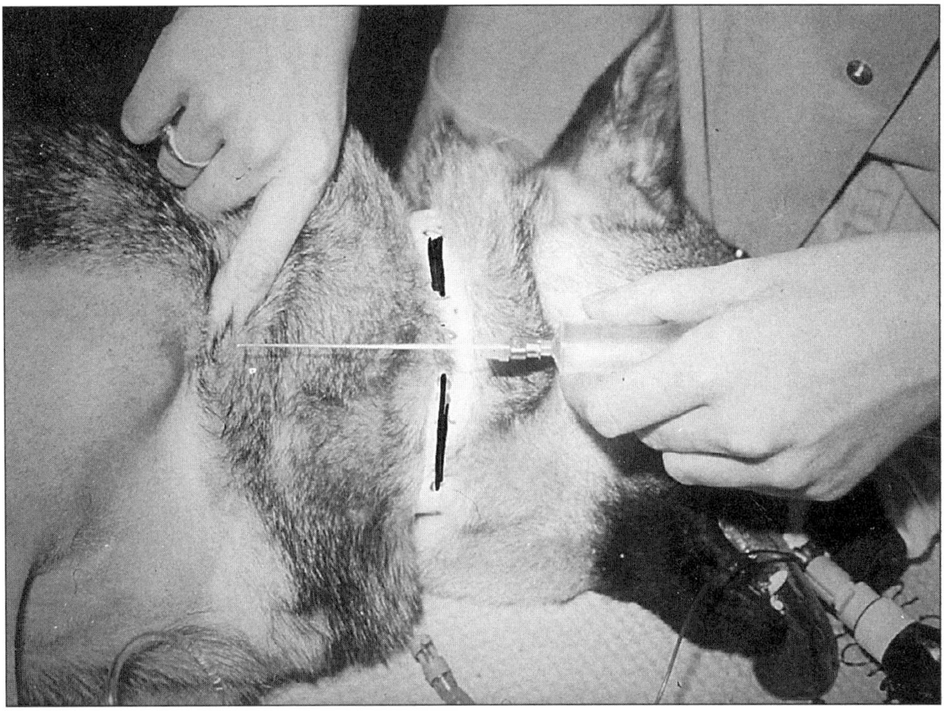

***Figure A-2***. *Performance of a brachial plexus block.*
***Figure A-2 A***. *The site for the brachial plexus block is clipped and prepped. A spinal needle is used in this dog. Notice the angle of the needle in reference to the scapulo-humeral joint, thoracic wall, and vertebral column. (Photograph courtesy of Dr. Elizabeth Martinez.)*

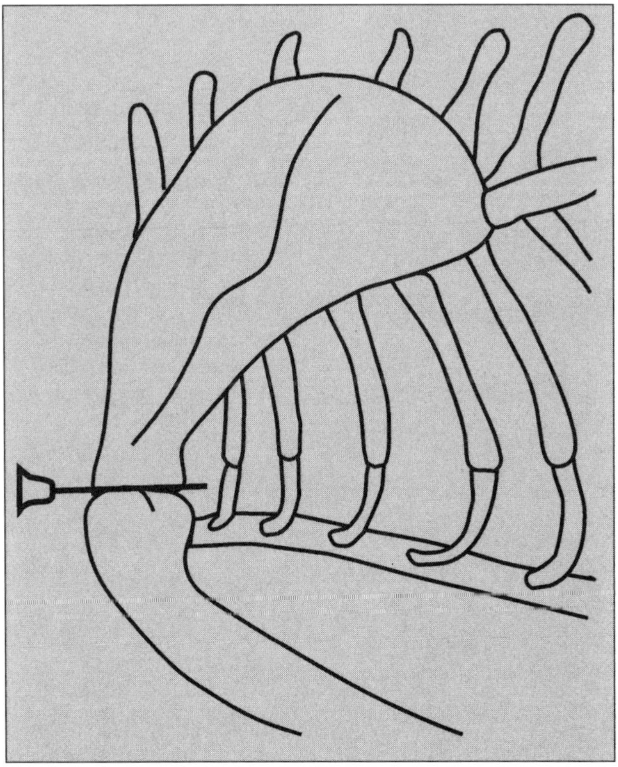

***Figure A-2 B***. *Note the placement of the needle: medial to the scapulo-humeral joint, lateral to the thoracic wall, toward the costochondral junction, and parallel to the vertebral column.*

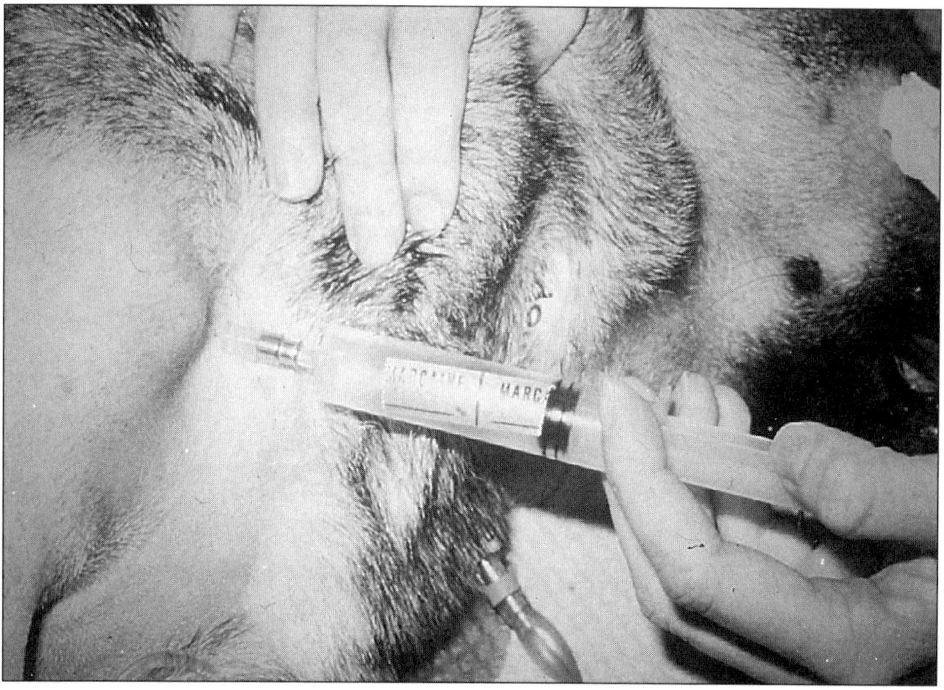

***Figure A-2 C.*** *The depression for needle placement is evident. Aspirate to assure that the needle has not been placed in a vessel; inject the appropriate drug as the needle is withdrawn. (Photograph courtesy of Dr. Elizabeth Martinez.)*

ensure that the needle is not in a vessel and inject slowly as the needle is withdrawn. The area from the foot up to the elbow should be desensitized.

## References


1. Pascoe PJ. Advantages and guidelines for using epidural drugs for analgesia. Vet Clin No Am: Sm An Prac 1992; 22:421–24.
2. Robinson EP. Perioperative and postoperative pain control in the dog and cat. In: Animal pain and its control. Proceedings 226 in conjunction with the Chapter of Anaesthetics and Intensive Care of the Australian College of Veterinary Scientists. Sydney: Post Graduate Committee in Veterinary Science University of Sydney, 1994:423–39.

# Appendix B Drugs and Sources

The drugs and sources provided are not the only ones available, but are meant to be a representation. Generally, the drugs and sources cited are the ones with which the author has had exposure. Always read the package insert for warnings and precautions.

**Acepromazine Maleate**

Trade name: Promace
Concentration: 10 mg/ml
How supplied: 50 ml/vial
Company: Fort Dodge Laboratories, Inc.
Fort Dodge, IA 50501

**Atipamezole HCl**

Trade name: Antisedan
Concentration: 5 mg/ml
How supplied: 10 ml/vial
Manufacturer: Orion Corporation
Espoo, Finland
Distributor: Pfizer Animal Health
New York, NY 10017

**Atropine**

Label name: Atropine Injectable
Concentration: 0.5 mg/ml*
How supplied: 50 ml/vial
Company: Fort Dodge Laboratories, Inc.
Fort Dodge, IA 50501

Label name: Atropine Sulfate
Concentration: 0.5 mg/ml
How supplied: 100 ml/vial
Company: Radix Laboratories, Inc.
Eau Claire, WI 54701

* Other concentrations are available.

**Bupivacaine Hydrochloride**

Trade name: Marcaine Hydrochloride
Concentration: 5 mg/ml*
How supplied: 10 ml/vial, 30 ml/vial, and 50 ml/vial
Company: Sanofi Winthrop Pharmaceuticals
New York, NY 10016

**Buprenorphine Hydrochloride**
**Schedule V**

Trade name: Buprenex Injectable
Concentration: 0.3 mg/ml
How supplied: 1 ml/ampule in a box of 5
Manufacturer: Reckitt & Coleman Products Ltd.
Hull, England HU87DS
Distributor: Reckitt & Coleman Pharmaceutical Inc.
Richmond, VA 23235

**Butorphanol**
**Schedule IV**

Trade name: Stadol
Concentration: 2 mg/ml*
How supplied: 10 ml/vial
Company: Apothecon
Princeton, NJ 08540

**Butorphanol Tartrate**

Trade name: Torbugesic-SA
Concentration: 2 mg/ml
How supplied: 10 ml/vial
Company: Fort Dodge Laboratories, Inc.
Fort Dodge, IA 50501

Trade name: Torbugesic
Concentration: 10 mg/ml
How supplied: 50 ml/vial
Company: Fort Dodge Laboratories, Inc.
Fort Dodge, IA 50501

Trade name: Torbutrol
Tablet size: 1 mg, 5 mg, 10 mg
How supplied: 100/bottle
Company: Fort Dodge Laboratories, Inc.
Fort Dodge, IA 50501

**Carprofen**

Trade name: Rimadyl
Caplet size: 25 mg, 75 mg, 100 mg
How supplied: 100, 250/bottle
Company: Pfizer Animal Health
Exton, PA 19341

* Other concentrations are available.

**Diazepam**
**Schedule IV**

Label name: Diazepam Injection, USP
Concentration: 5 mg/ml
How supplied: 10 ml/vial
Company: Steris Laboratories, Inc.
Phoenix, AZ 85043

**Etomidate**

Trade name: Amidate
Concentration: 2 mg/ml
How supplied: 20 ml/ampule
Company: Abbott Laboratories
North Chicago, IL 60064

Label name: Etomidate
Concentration: 2 mg/ml
How supplied: 20 ml vial
Manufactured by: Ben Venue Laboratories, Inc.
Bedford, OH 44146, for
Bedford Laboratories
Bedford, OH 44146

**Fentanyl IV**
**Schedule II**

Label name: Fentanyl Citrate Injection, USP
Concentration: 50 μg/ml
How supplied: 2 ml/ampule, 10 ampules
Company: Abbott Laboratories
North Chicago, IL 60064

**Fentanyl Transdermal System**
**Schedule II**

Trade name: Duragesic
Patch size: 25 μg/h, 50 μg/h, 75 μg/h, 100 μg/h
Manufacturer: ALZA Corporation
Palo Alto, CA 94304
Distributor: Janssen Pharmaceutica, Inc.
Titusville, NJ 08560

**Flumazenil**

Trade name: Romazicon
Concentration: 0.1 mg/ml
How supplied: 5 ml, 10 ml vials
Company: Roche Diagnostic Systems
Somerville, NJ 08876-3771

**Flunixin Meglumine**

Trade name: Banamine Solution
Concentration: 50 mg/ml
How supplied: 50 ml, 100 ml vials
Company: Schering-Plough Animal Health
Kenilworth, NJ 07033

**Glycopyrrolate**

Trade name: Robinul-V
Concentration: 0.2 mg/ml
How supplied: 20 ml/vial
Company: Fort Dodge Laboratories, Inc.
Fort Dodge, IA 50501

**Ketamine HCl**

Trade name: Ketaset
Concentration: 100 mg/ml
How supplied: 10 ml/vial
Company: Fort Dodge Laboratories, Inc.
Fort Dodge, IA 50501

**Ketoprofen**

Trade name: Ketofen
Concentration: 100 mg/ml
How supplied: 50 ml, 100 ml vials
Company: Fort Dodge Laboratories
Fort Dodge, IA 50501

Trade name: Orudis
How supplied: 25 mg, 50 mg capsules, 100/bottle, 75 mg capsules, 100 or 500/bottle
Company: Wyeth-Ayerst
Philadelphia, PA 19101

Trade name: Oruvail
Size: 100 mg, 150 mg, 200 mg extended release capsules
How supplied: 100/bottle
Company: Wyeth-Ayerst
Philadelphia, PA 19101

**Ketorolac Tromethamine**

Trade name: Toradol
How supplied: Tubex syringes
15 mg: 15 mg/ml
30 mg: 30 mg/ml
60 mg: 30 mg/ml
Manufacturer: Wyeth Laboratories
Philadelphia, PA 19101
Distributor: Syntex Laboratories
Palo Alto, CA 94304

Trade name: Toradol
Tablet size: 10 mg
How supplied: 100/bottle
Company: Syntex Laboratories
Palo Alto, CA 94304

**Lidocaine**

Trade name: Xylocaine
Concentration: 20 mg/ml
How supplied: 20 ml/vial
Company: Astra Labs, Inc.
Westborough, MA 01581

Trade name: Lidocaine HCL 2%
Concentration: 20 mg/ml
How supplied: 100 ml/vial
Company: Western Veterinary Supply, Inc.
Portersville, CA 93257

Trade name: Emla cream
Concentration: lidocaine 2.5% and prilocaine 2.5%
How supplied: 5 g tube, box of 1 or 5; 30 g tube, box of 1
Manufacturer: Astra Pharm.
Sodertalje, Sweden
Distributor: Astra USA, Inc.
Westborough, MA 01581

**Meclofenamate**

Trade name: Arquel
Tablet size: 10 mg, 20 mg
How supplied: 500/bottle
Company: Fort Dodge Laboratories
Fort Dodge, IA 50501

**Medetomidine HCl**

Trade name: Domitor
Concentration: 1 mg/ml
How supplied: 10 ml/vial
Manufacturer: Orion Corporation
Espoo, Finland
Distributor: Pfizer Animal Health
New York, NY 10017

**Meperidine HCl**
**Schedule II**

Trade name: Demerol
Concentration: 50 mg/ml*
How supplied: 30 ml/vial
Distributor: Sanofi Winthrop Pharmaceuticals
New York, NY 10016

**Methohexital Sodium**
**Schedule IV**

Trade name: Brevital
How supplied: 500 mg/vial in a 50 ml multidose vial
Company: Eli Lilly and Company
Indianapolis, IN 46285

**Morphine**
**Schedule II**

Trade name: Duramorph (Preservative Free)
Concentration: 0.5 mg/ml
How supplied: 10 ml/ampule
Company: Elkins-Sinn, Inc.
Cherry Hill, NJ 08003-4099

Trade name: Morphine Sulfate
Concentration: 15 mg/ml*
How supplied: 20 ml/vial
Company: Elkins-Sinn, Inc.
Cherry Hill, NJ 08003-4099

**Nalbuphine HCl**

Trade name: Nubain
Concentration: 20 mg/ml*
How supplied: 10 ml/vial
Company: DuPont Merck Pharma
Manati, Puerto Rico 00674

* Other concentrations are available.

**Naloxone**

Trade name: Narcan
Concentration: 0.4 mg/ml
How supplied: 10 ml/vial
Company: DuPont Merck Pharma
Manati, Puerto Rico 00674

**Oxymorphone HCl**
**Schedule II**

Trade name: Numorphan
Concentration: 1.5 mg/ml*
How supplied: 10 ml/vial
Company: DuPont Merck Pharma
Manati, Puerto Rico 00674

**Pentazocine Lactate**
**Schedule IV**

Trade name: Talwin
Concentration: 30 mg/ml
How supplied: 10 ml/vial
Company: Sanofi Winthrop
New York, NY 10016

**Propofol**

Trade name: Diprivan
Concentration: 10 mg/ml
How supplied: 20 ml ampule, 50 & 100 ml vial
Manufacturer: Zeneca S.P.A.
Distributor: Zeneca Pharmaceuticals
Wilmington, DE 19850-5437

Trade name: Rapinovet
Concentration: 10 mg/ml
How supplied: 20 ml ampule
Distributor: Mallinkrodt Veterinary, Inc.
Mundelein, IL 60060

**Thiopental**
**Schedule III**

Trade name: Veterinary Pentothal
How supplied: 5% (Reconstituted in 100 ml)
5 g powder
Company: Abbott Laboratories
North Chicago, IL 60064

* Other concentrations are available.

**Tiletamine HCl–Zolazepam HCl**
**Schedule III**

Trade name: Telazol
Concentration: 100 mg/ml (when reconstituted)
How supplied: 5 ml/vial
Manufacturer: Elkins-Sinn Inc.
Cherry Hill, NJ 08003-4099
Distributor: Fort Dodge Laboratories, Inc.
Fort Dodge, IA 50501

**Tolazoline HCl**

Trade name: Priscoline HCl
Concentration: 25 mg/ml
How supplied: 4 ml/ampule
Manufacturer: Ciba-Giegy Limited
Basle, Switzerland
Distributor: Ciba Geigy Corporation
Summit, NJ 07901

Trade name: Tolazine
Concentration: 100 mg/ml
How supplied: 100 ml/vial
Distributor: Lloyd Laboratories
Shenandoah, IA 51601

**Xylazine HCl**

Trade name: Rompun SA
Concentration: 20 mg/ml
How supplied: 20 ml/vial
Company: Miles Inc.
Shawnee Mission, KS 66201

Trade name: Rompun
Concentration: 100 mg/ml
How supplied: 50 ml/vial
Company: Bayer Corporation
Shawnee Mission, KS 66201

**Yohimbine**

Trade name: Yobine
Concentration: 2 mg/ml
How supplied: 20 ml/vial
Distributor: Lloyd Laboratories
Shenandoah, IA 51601

# Index

# About the Author

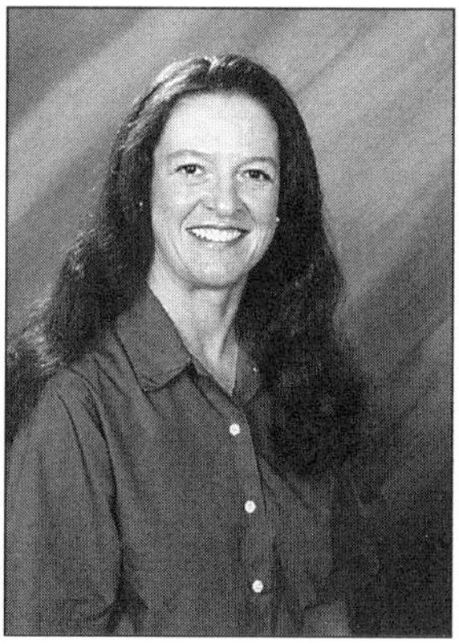

Gwendolyn Light Carroll, MS, DVM, is an assistant professor of anesthesiology at Texas A&M University. Dr. Carroll received an AB in bio-psychology (animal behavior) from Vassar College and an MS in animal science with a major in genetics (the heritability of the stress response in beef cattle) from the University of Tennessee. She also received her veterinary degree from the University of Tennessee. Dr. Carroll was a small animal practitioner for 8 years before returning to the University of North Carolina for a post doctoral fellowship in postoperative analgesia. At the conclusion of her fellowship, she pursued her interest in postoperative analgesia through a residency in anesthesiology at the University of North Carolina. The common thread through her education, training, research, and practice has been an enduring interest in animal behavior and well-being. She currently lives with her husband Tim Carroll and two red tabby domestic short hair cats, Dennis and DJ.